I Can Make You HOT!

I Can Make You HOT!

THE SUPERMODEL DIET

Kelly Killoren Bensimon

St. Martin's Press ✻ New York

www.stmartins.com

Design by Richard Oriolo
Food photography by Jerrit Clark

ISBN 978-1-250-00556-4 (hardcover)
ISBN 978-1-4668-0239-1 (e-book)

First Edition: April 2012

10 9 8 7 6 5 4 3 2 1

To my beautiful girls, who inspire me to be the best woman and most energetic mom I can be. I don't want to miss out on anything. I love you.

contents

acknowledgments

I'd like to take a minute to thank everyone who worked tirelessly on this book, who laughed with me, and who helped me achieve all of those "ah ha" moments you don't ever think you will have writing a book, but inevitably do.

To Jill Zarin who called Steve Cohen and said, "This girl has a great book in her."

To St. Martin's Press for believing in me; to Steve Cohen for meeting me over the phone and deciding in less than five minutes that I needed to meet with his editors, and for believing in me; to Elizabeth Beier, who offered me a book deal in less than twenty-four hours, and recognized an authentic voice when she heard it; and to John Murphy, who laughs at all my jokes and gets why you need to treat your body like a Ferrari.

To Andrea Barzvi, my agent from ICM, who signed her deal with me while she was weeks pregnant (I can't imagine talking diet or food when I was pregnant; thank you, Andrea).

To Lauren Zalaznick, who saw me as more than a girl who looks like "someone" and gave me an entirely new life that makes it possible for me to provide for my girls.

A special thank-you to Christian Barcellos, who, after trying to put me on a TV show with Tim Gunn, pulled me aside to ask if I'd help him out with the *Real Housewives of New York City*. He told me I'd have a blast with the show. I never knew that one altercation with one stranger could put a show on the map. Thank you, Christian, for believing in me, and for helping me define who I am and what I love, one mistake at a time. Clearly reality TV bites, but it doesn't sting.

To Andy Cohen, who believed in me for many seasons of the *Real Housewives of New York City*.

To Seth Levine, who is an amazing chef and has seen me raw, real, and uncensored, and who has taught me how to make my food taste *great* in less than three tries.

To my second assistant, Melissa Thompson, who threw

herself into this book with me and went over it line by line to make sure everything was along the lines of KKBfit.

To Alexa Rea, who helped me research a lot of facts and apply them to my diet doctrine.

To my best friend, Leah McCloskey, who has cooked for me many times and always told me to be proud of who I am.

To my amazing glam squad, Bradley Irion and Quinn Murphy, who always make me look so amazing, even when I haven't felt good about myself.

To Fernando Romano, who has been like a father to me in New York City and has taken care of all my finances.

To my sister and brother, who laughed at me when I cooked for them (I would have cried if I were the one tasting that food). To my sister-in-law, Mimi, who encouraged my sister's idea to write a book about living well and eating well. Here's your book. I did it for you.

To Carol Goll for taking me to ICM and seeing me as a household name.

To *Shape* magazine and Tara Kraft for their amazing September 2011 cover, which foreshadowed the ideas in *I Can Make You Hot!*

To Tom Scott, Dan Honan, Chris Connors, and everyone at Plum TV for forecasting a future career for me. *Behind the Hedges* allowed me to show the allure and what I admire about amazing vacation destinations and talented people.

To Samantha Marcus Yanks, who created the InShape column in *Hamptons* magazine for me to explore what to do, what to wear, and where to go to enjoy a healthful lifestyle in the Hamptons.

To the coaches for all of my sports, and to anyone who ever ran with me, during any marathon, or even saw me on the street and said "hello" while running.

And to Professor Alan Ziegler from Columbia University, who inspired me to write about what I know and love. I am forever grateful.

I'd like especially to thank Eric Ripert for always offering to open up his kitchen to me and for trying to encourage me to cook, and hopefully cook well. He taught me a valuable lesson about cooking, that making food for those you love is a luxury, and that is always how I have thought about it. Thank you, Eric, for your amazing dishes and for feeding me while I was attending Columbia. Your talent and love for good food is infectious.

Special thanks to Judy Kern, my amazing writer, who made healthy living so much fun and inspired me to channel my passion and hard work into words, not be intimidated, and to enjoy the process.

To Jami Kandel, who has promoted and saved me from my own big mouth many times. Her vision of who I am and what I'm good at has always been true to my core and filled with integrity.

To my parents, who traveled with me all over the world and not only expanded my horizons but exposed me to the finest cuisine.

A special thanks to my assistant, Stephanie Posner, who came in at the last minute and encouraged me to hone my skills and explore what I love with no boundaries.

And last but not least I'd like to dedicate a special thank-you to my former assistant, Kim Thompson, who worked tirelessly with me and never lost track of what was in our future. She always admired the way I ate and lived my life and encouraged me to expose to the world a new kind of eating.

foreword

I've known Kelly a long time. My kids and I call her "KellyBensimon," one happy word all run together. Whenever she comes over with her kids in the Hamptons, everyone runs around saying "KellyBensimon is here!" Yes, her name is one word in our house. Even my brother, RevRun and his wife, Justine, love KellyBensimon. Every time I see her with her kids, she reminds me what deep personal satisfaction is. Kelly is a great mother and is constantly instilling strong principals in her daughters. In my opinion, that's the essence of being HOT. Kelly is *smokin'*.

I met her when she was nineteen years old with director Brett Ratner. No one forgets meeting Kelly for the first time. Her genuine energy is something most people wish to have. Her beauty truly comes from within, and her clear internal compass and well-balanced lifestyle is what makes her an arbiter for what's hot. She has always had her own individual road map and is one of those people who beats to their own drum. Many are amazed by her leaps of faith and courage, which are products of her sustainable soul. And back to that energy! I used to think: If we could only package it. And now Kelly has!

Right after she was married in 1997, Kelly asked me to help her with a charity for Hale House, a center in Harlem that sheltered children of drug addicts who were born with HIV. Kelly had a clever idea and went for it, despite a lot of criticism. She asked celebs to autograph jeans, which she then sold as art to raise money. I had no idea before that moment that she was so creative in her drive for helping others. It was impressive to say the least.

To me, she's always been the same clever, crazy Kelly-Bensimon. She was a model, of course—she still looks like a model, acts like a model, walks like a model, and dresses like a model, but her style sense doesn't come from her line of work. Instead, it's an outward manifestation of knowing and staying true to herself, sans stylists and photographers. KellyBensimon dresses like KellyBensimon.

There's no secret to Kelly's body. She's always been on the path to pursue constant well-being: 25 percent exercise, 25 percent eating well, and 100 percent loving life. Kelly always made it her life choice to be healthy, regardless of any circumstances. She learned good habits from modeling, but come on—those legs are genetic! No yoga pose on the planet is going to make legs look like that, even if you can tap her spirit and her energy by using the advice in this book. I know she is also very active and ran the New York City marathon, all over the Hamptons, and loves riding horses. She has more energy than any person her age I've ever met—she is twenty-four, isn't she?

That's a testament not only to what Kelly puts in her body but also to her spirit. You can't be happy and healthy without paying attention to your spirit as well as your body. Kelly has always been very comfortable and happy with who she is, and no one will deny that.

That's the one thing about Kelly that people want—part of her happiness. How do I get her real, inherent happiness? Happiness isn't something you are handed, but it's something you have to be aware of on a daily basis and work at constantly. Gold, shiny objects do not act as incentives in the pursuit of happiness. Kelly knows that her happiness is justified by the life she wants for herself and her kids, and is reflected by that genuine smile you can't wipe off her face. When you see it firsthand, you just know it comes from an inherently grounded place. You can't take her happiness, but she'll give you the shirt off her back—just don't expect her to be on time for the exchange.

She can't transform anyone into a rock star, but she can show you how to rock—what you do with it is *your* choice. That's KellyBensimon. Her journey is just starting. If the past is a prologue, we are in for a good ride.

—RUSSELL SIMMONS, 2012

I Can
Make You
HOT!

Introduction:
What's HOT and What's Not

How do you get HOT? Hot to me is not predicated on a diet but on the way you choose to live your life—by choosing Healthy Options Today, and tomorrow, and every day. My HOT philosophy is based on a high-energy way of eating and living. Its foundation is a back-to-basics style of eating all food groups with an emphasis on eating smart proteins and smart carbs that provide all the energy I need to be an active participant in life. Just as I want you to challenge your mind with smart information, I want you to challenge your body. I want you to see it all, do it all, and enjoy it all. I'm not a doctor or an expert of any kind. I'm just a mom who was a teenage competitive swimmer and a model, who has lost fifty pounds twice, has run the New York City Marathon, graced the covers of *Playboy* at forty-one and *Shape* at forty-three years old, and who has struggled with size issues for much of her adult life. Was I overweight as a child? No. Let's just say that I was never one of those tiny, cute blonde girls who guys named their hamsters after, and I was aware of the difference between those girls and me.

My daily routine requires endurance and stamina. When I'm not working and raising my tween girls on my own, I've done everything—appear on a television show with a group of women who seem to fight all day, edit a fashion magazine, work on my various businesses, and write. . . . So I need to be well fed and on my game every day.

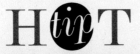

Chase a healthy lifestyle with a vengeance—the way you'd chase a hot guy (or girl).

In this book I'm going to clue you in on all the tricks I've learned from a variety of experts that I use myself. I want you to be the best you—happy, attractive, shapely, interested, interesting, and, most of all, feeling smokin' HOT. Truthfully, you are already hot. You know it and I know it. But everyone has good days and bad days. My job with this book is to help you maximize the good days and ultimately make them a way of life.

When I was trying to come up with a title for this book, I kept asking myself how I would define what I love. "HOT" is the word that best describes what I love, and it's not a word I throw around lightly. "HOT" is attractive, unique, and first-rate—never mediocre. Avril Lavigne made a video called "HOT." There are "HOT" issues of all my favorite magazines. Hotmail.com was given that name to indicate that it was the best e-mail service, and www.urbandictionary.com, whose definitions are created by their readers, defines "hot" as (among other things) *attractive*, *the best*, and *someone who makes you wish you had a pause button when they walk by because you don't want that moment to end*. (I want you to feel like that "someone.") Health, wellness, and fitness are always hot topics. "HOT" may be a buzzword but it's also how I describe the best there is and the best you can be. I've used the words "smokin' hot" for everything from a killer chicken wing red sauce to a coveted couture gown.

The term started to take on meaning for me while I was writing *American Style*. In 1978 Hubert de Givenchy recognized our innovative talents by telling the American designers who came to Paris with jeans, camp-style shirts, and a fresh new take on fashion that Americans were "cool." HOT is cool! And after researching all the people with different body shapes who have worn the bikini since the '50s for *The Bikini Book*, I finally started to define what was smokin' HOT to me. I love the pioneer, the person who's proud, has a lot of integrity, who works hard and loves harder. The one who makes the most fabulous handbag or who has vital information to share—these are the people I find HOT.

So how do you get HOT? By eating well, sleeping well, and exercising daily. By following this lifestyle, you will be an active participant in your own life and ultimately make good decisions. I didn't always make good decisions for myself. You're not going to believe me, but I've considered myself fat. And I could have stayed fat. Instead I decided to make different decisions every single day, because for me there really isn't any alternative.

Is skinny hot? Naturally skinny is hot. Starving yourself in order to change your natural body type in order to get skinny is *not* hot. I'm not advocating that everyone weigh 104 pounds. If you are starving or missing meals, you are focusing on food, not on life. But, at the other end of the spectrum, being overweight or obese is certainly not hot; it's just plain unhealthy. According to the most recent statistics more than 30 percent of Americans are obese. In France it's 9.4 percent; in Italy it's 8.5. There's no reason for that. Americans have all the same food choices available to us; we just need to make the right ones so that we can be as healthy as possible for our own body types.

For me, the ultimate HOT girl is the nineteenth-century Gibson girl. As created by Charles Dana Gibson, she was the original pinup, a shapely personification of the new all-American girl. She swam in the ocean wearing culottes and loved every minute of it. She was (is!) cool, curvy, and the guys want to be around her because she's happy, healthy, athletic, and having a lot of fun. She's free to go anywhere and do anything she wants without worrying about having every hair in place or ruining her clothes. An example of a modern Gibson girl is Bethany Hamilton, the young surfer who lost an arm in a shark attack and didn't let it stop her from pursuing a sport she loves. She's smokin' HOT.

So, how did I arrive at this definition? It's actually taken a long time, with ups and downs (emotionally and physically) along the way. I was always a very active child, and even more so when I became a competitive swimmer in my early teens. I was always tall, but I was also athletic, and being tall was never a problem for me. In fact, the boys I grew up with were mostly athletic—that's just how we grow them in the Midwest.

At fifteen, I entered a national model search contest in *Seventeen* magazine. People had been telling me that I should model, so when I found the contest I decided I might as well enter and see if they were right. I didn't win, but I was one of the runners-up. I then entered another contest sponsored by *Teen* magazine, and this time I was runner-up to one of those teeny blonde girls. The next contest I entered was sponsored by Elite Model Management. By that time I was sixteen and was again runner-up—this time to Cindy Crawford. The agency invited us both to come to New York, where they measured, weighed, and put us through a routine that was like taking a physical to join the army. In the end, what the people at the agency who hired me found beautiful about me—my smile, my inner happiness, and healthful attitude—they subsequently tried to take away by telling me, all day every day, that I had to lose ten pounds. I was 5 foot 10 and weighed a healthy, muscular 140 pounds. They wanted me to be a skinny 130. Those ten pounds became my nemesis. For the first time in my life I hated the way I looked. I suddenly felt "big" and ungainly.

I was definitely in danger of developing an eating disorder, and what saved me during those years was running. I ran almost every day, mainly to keep my weight down and my spirits high. I ran, even when everyone else was telling me what I should do to look better. My self-esteem was at a low point, but running always made me feel good physically.

It all came to a head when I was pregnant with my first daughter. Most people feel confident and settled when they get pregnant, but I was the wife of a famous fashion photographer who was also the international creative director of *Elle* and worked with supermodels every day. There I was tipping the scales at 190 and surrounded by models who were desperate to get thinner as I was getting wider. I was alone on "Pregnancy Island" and I felt awkward, unfulfilled. I was wearing men's shirts when everyone around me was talking about hot abs on supermodels.

In case you think I shouldn't have been feeling so sorry for myself, I hasten to say that I've been privileged to know and work with some pretty amazing people, and one of them came to my rescue and helped snap me out of the pregnancy blues. Calvin Klein said he wanted to make me a few dresses and invited me to come in for a fitting. Before we got started, I was sitting across from him in his office when out of nowhere I started to tear up. I was overwhelmed by my ever-widening waistline, hormonally challenged and scared about being a new mom in the modeling world, and Calvin was not only a designer but also a dad. I knew he would understand what I was feeling.

He was totally focused on me while his staff waved their

hands, desperately trying to get his attention. Calvin Klein's new ad campaign featured what looked like teenage models in provocative positions. The world was offended and upset, but Calvin knew the campaign would sell more underwear and jeans than a pretty girl any day. He is a brilliant designer and a marketing maverick. But I digress. The irony, which was lost on me at the time, is that while I was crying about being wide he was in the process of defending an infamous, industry-changing ad campaign featuring skinny underage kids. His staff raced him out the back door while a team of men and women dressed entirely in black came in to take my measurements. When they asked me my size, I said "wide."

A few weeks later a black garment bag arrived with a long purple slip dress cut on the bias for maximum growth potential, a low-cut black sheath dress, and a long riding-style coat. I realized then that he wanted me to have clothes that would allow me to love the way I looked throughout my pregnancy. Thank you, Calvin Klein, for taking me from wide to HOT. Reflecting back, I wish I'd been able to recognize then, as I do now, that pregnancy is smokin' HOT.

It wasn't until after I'd had my two daughters that my perspective started to shift. Instead of being focused on my waist size, I began to focus on my girls and my writing. My career was starting to blossom, and possibilities I had never even imagined began to arise. I was thinking about what could be, not about what I wanted to change about me. I had regained my inner confidence, which ultimately led to the ending of my marriage. My divorce from Gilles had nothing to do with him and everything to do with where I was in my own life. To this day, we have a healthy and happy relationship.

So, whatever you're going through or have been through in terms of your health and self-esteem, I've been there. I've tried every diet (*die* with a *t*), every fast, and every juice cleanse—and each time I've gone right back to my real body weight, which I now love no matter what anyone says. If I could do that, if I could endure all the pressure and come out the other side, so can you.

I don't want to pretend that I'm "just like you." To do that would be disingenuous, and you wouldn't believe me anyway. But I may be more like you than you think. My hair may look ready for Victoria's Secret, but my values are still Midwestern. I'm raising two daughters, I cook for them and for myself (and, no, I don't have a personal chef—except when my kids do the cooking), and I want to instill in them the Midwestern values I grew up with. When I joined the cast of *Real Housewives of New York City*, fans of the program and my Twitter followers asked me what I do to stay fit, which made me realize that I do have information to share and that people really do want to know. To answer all their questions I created the hashtag #KKBfit, which has since become the inspiration for this book.

Everyone has the capacity to be HOT. I don't have any special DNA that makes me hotter than the next woman. But I have learned lessons and acquired a few tricks that will help you to gain the confidence to be your absolute hottest. And, after all, why wouldn't you want to be HOT? What's the alternative? Being "not so hot"?

For a long time I was reluctant to share my weight-loss stories. I was flattered that anyone would be interested in how I eat and live, but I'm basically shy (believe it or not), and I also didn't really think people would believe me. I thought they'd just look at me as I am now and assume I was "born that way." The truth is that I've worked hard to create the balance I believe is the only way to be healthy, happy, and ultimately HOT. I wanted to dispel the mistaken idea that skinny is hot, and overexercised is healthy.

I've been photographed as a skinny bag of anxiety-starved bones after Season 3 of the *Real Housewives of New York City*. I never in a million years thought I'd become the victim of a story line. But the press went to town with an assumption, and I was a mess as a result: insecure, nervous, and scared. To combat all the negativity, I ate well, even though I kept getting skinnier, and I didn't give up. I continued eating well, loving my kids, family, and friends, sleeping well, and smiling whenever I could to anyone, anywhere.

During Season 4, I was so grounded and felt so comfortable and proud of myself that I became the voice of reason on the show. Who would have thought I'd survive the wrath of mean girls? So, if you're going through a divorce, being sued, or having your integrity defamed by strangers on national television, I've been there and I survived while the whole world watched me. Today, I'm confident enough to tell my story. Sometimes in life you have to endure a speed bump. I love those who survive and do it looking HOT. We make our own choices about how to deal with adversity, so my advice is, any time you fall victim to bad thoughts, eat some dehydrated fruit, drink a glass of raspberry-infused lemonade, take a spin on your bicycle, smile all the way through life, and never for a moment think you are alone because I'm doing the same thing, probably on the exact same day you are.

So let's get HOT together, day-by-day, step-by-step, meal-by-meal, by eating well, sleeping well, feeling good, and having fun. I've divided this book into seven days, with something different to focus on and work on each day. I urge you to make notes as you go along, either in the book itself or, if writing in a book is anathema to you, in a little notebook to use as your own personal guide. Jotting down ideas as they pop into your head is the best way to process them and be sure that they don't leave again before you've had a chance to commit them to long-term memory. Then, if you've made a mistake, when you go back and see it there on paper, you'll remind yourself not to do it again. Or, as I like to say, you'll avoid getting bitten by the same food dog twice! And, conversely, if something really worked for you, you'll remember to do it again—and again, until it becomes part of your normal, everyday lifestyle. It isn't hard. In fact, my plan is very simple:

1. **Exercise every day. No excuses.**
2. **Make healthy food choices and eat well six days a week.**
3. **Make Sunday your Funday and eat whatever you want. If you've been making good choices and moving your body the other six days, you get to "fall off the wagon" once a week.**

By the time you've read through the book, you'll have a whole new plan for eating and living well for the rest of your life. I think you'll be surprised to learn that some of the foods you thought you should *never* eat (such as starchy carbs and sugar) are actually the ones you should be eating every day. I might as well admit it right now: I eat carbs and sugar all the time. I never deny myself rice or sweets, but I try to make good carb choices, and I don't overdo. Every single time I've tried to do something different, such as give up carbs or give up meat, my body rebelled. Your body has a voice (and I don't mean your stomach grumbling); you just need to listen to the signals it's sending and respond appropriately.

I'm going to be sharing with you how to do what I do, and I can guarantee that if you follow my life plan you *will* be *smokin' HOT* from your head to your toes and from your heart to your skin, inside and out!

Monday: Make a List–Plan and Prepare!

To me, living well is the only option. What, after all, is the only alternative? Living badly? Who aspires to living badly? I want you to live well, and that's going to take some planning.

What are your goals for yourself? If you're going to make changes in your life, you need to have a plan, you need to prepare, and you need to take the time to get it right—so that you don't wind up wasting your time. This is my plan, and from now on it's going to be yours. Monday is going to be the day you make a HOT plan and prepare for the rest of your week. Let's get started together!

What are you going to be eating this week? I know we haven't talked about specific meals yet (we'll be doing that on Wednesday). For now, you just need to know that planning your meals in advance and shopping for the foods you're going to need for the rest of the week will help to keep you on track. If what you need or want to eat isn't there when you want it, you're likely to substitute something a lot less healthy and satisfying just because it's staring you in the face.

Another positive side effect of this is that once you've finished your food shopping you'll know how much money you have left over to spend on other things. And you're less likely to buy things you don't really need—so you might have some extra cash for a pedicure. This isn't just about budgeting your food; it's about budgeting your life.

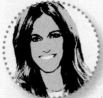

Kelly's Cardinal Rule

This is not something you don't know, but—never go shopping when you're hungry. That's when you're most likely to make bad choices and find yourself finishing a whole bag of Peanut M&M's while you're surfing the vegetable aisle. You don't want to be that person who is snacking while you're shopping. That's not hot—period.

Staples I keep in my house

SNACKS

Almonds

Dehydrated mangos, blueberries, pineapple

Unbuttered, unsalted popcorn

Kale chips

Organic fruit snacks

Olives

Wasabi-roasted green peas

Yogurt-covered goji berries

BREADS, CEREALS, FLOUR, AND GRAINS

Bran and whole wheat cereals

Brown and white rice

Cornbread mix

Lentils

Organic brownie mix

Pancake mix

Rice crackers

Taco shells

Whole grain croutons

Whole wheat pasta

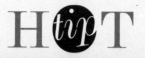

I'm not a big fan of nuts in general, but I do love almonds, and they have many health benefits. They're packed with nutrients and monounsaturated fats that help keep your heart healthy.

Olives may be little balls of fat, but they're full of health-promoting, omega-9 monounsaturated fatty acids as well as vitamin E and flavonoids, which are potent antioxidants. Plus, black olives have more iron than any other food and there is research to show that olives and olive oil may be effective in the prevention and treatment of arthritis, asthma, and some types of cancer. They also satisfy your need for salt and combat cravings.

FRUITS AND VEGETABLES

Avocado

Baby carrots

Bananas

Blueberries

Celery

Cherry tomatoes

Edamame (fresh soy beans)

Frozen peas

Frozen spinach

Mixed salad greens

Oranges

Snow peas

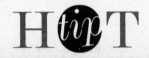

Dehydrated snow peas are the new edamame.

Try different kinds of milk for different flavors. See which ones you like best.

BEVERAGES

Bottled water

Unsweetened coconut milk/almond milk/whole cow's milk/soy milk/vanilla soy milk

Diet Coke (Yes, I drink Diet Coke but I don't drink gallons of it every day, and neither should you!)

Lemonade

Organic chamomile with lavender tea

Peppermint tea

Pure white green tea

Coffee

Beer

Red wine

Tequila (my favorite is Patrón)

Vodka

White wine (I like Santa Margherita's pinot grigio)

DAIRY PRODUCTS

Butter

Eggs

Mozzarella cheese

Parmesan cheese

Yogurt

OTHER

Canned tuna, packed in water

Cinnamon, ground

Crushed red pepper flakes

Lavender-lemon pepper

Miso soup

Organic nonstick
cooking spray

Olive oil

Sugar

Sea salt

Truffle salt

Truffle oil

H tip T

I like using sea salt instead of regular salt because sea salt has more flavor and is more concentrated so you can use less of it to get the same taste.

Vodka sauce (I use Newman's Own because it's tasty and the company is a great charity organization—my two favorite things.)

h⊙t button issue

Many "diet" books will tell you not to drink because alcohol has empty calories and also lowers your inhibitions so that you're less likely to make good food choices.

Personally, I do drink beer, wine, and other alcoholic beverages. In fact, I love mixed drinks—particularly anything that comes with an umbrella—but not every day. When I was younger, I didn't drink beer. I didn't like it, and even one beer was too filling for me. My friends from Lake Geneva, Wisconsin, used to drink Old Style when we went to Chuck's, a local bar in Fontana, but I always drank soda. I probably drank a liter of soda every Saturday night. No wonder I was so energized!

Even later, in my twenties, I didn't really drink at all. I was modeling, traveling around the world, and attending Columbia University, all at the same time. I barely had any "me time," let alone bar time. Studying and partying don't mix.

After I gave birth to my first daughter, my doctor told me that my breast milk would flow more easily if I drank a dark beer every day. Since I'm Irish, I went with Guinness. That's when it started; my taste buds changed, and it was actually beneficial to me. Once I stopped breastfeeding I started to run more consistently again. Beer was already in my diet, and it also was refreshing and gave me carbs after my daily runs.

Do I encourage you to sit back and down a six-pack by yourself? Hardly! I don't drink beer (or any other alcohol) every day. Beer and I are now acquaintances, but not best friends. I don't lie around in front of the TV with a beer bottle on my belly. Everything with me is in moderation (except for how I love). No one ever looks HOT when they're drunk—even if they think they do—but if you don't have issues with alcohol, drink really good beer, wine, and alcohol. Bad alcohol leads to bad hangovers. And always, always, drink responsibly.

According to Forbes.com: "A vast number of studies show that moderate consumption of alcohol, including beer, may reduce the risk of heart disease—consistently the No. 1 cause of death in the United States. A 2006 study led by researchers at Beth Israel Deaconess Medical Center and the Harvard School of Public Health found that, among men with healthy lifestyles, those who consumed moderate amounts of alcohol had a 40 to 60% reduced risk of heart attack compared with heart healthy men who abstained." You heard it here.

And I read in the *New York Post* that Heidi Klum, ex-Victoria's Secret model and mother of four, runs four miles a day and drinks beer. If it's good enough for a former supermodel and for Forbes.com, it's good enough for me.

Interestingly, I've found that since I started taking care of my body and feeding it well, my metabolism works so efficiently that I can drink alcohol and metabolize it faster than most people. If you want to drink, my advice is to eat better and exercise!

H*tip*T

I firmly believe that bland food makes you fat. When food is really tasty, you're satisfied with less, so what you want is food so flavorful that you want to eat it slowly and savor every bite. Your taste buds will be in gastronomic heaven after just a few bites.

One way to get more of that sultry savory taste is to use truffle oil as a flavor enhancer. I love it on pasta, eggs, meat, and fish. Seth Levine, who appeared on Season 5 of Gordon Ramsay's hit television show, *Hell's Kitchen,* gave me some insight on truffles and how to use truffle oil. According to Seth, white truffles are more exotic and more expensive than black, are gathered during the summer only in France and Spain, and are mainly used in dishes during the fall months. Black truffles are more common and can be found in Oregon, Canada, and all over Europe throughout the year.

Truffle oil is so full of concentrated flavor that a little goes a very long way. Put a few drops on your salad or on a pizza. Just never add it until your food has finished cooking. Subjecting the oil to heat kills the truffle flavor. What a waste of deliciousness!

Think and Plan!

When you shop for clothes you probably have a budget. Think of food shopping the way you think of shopping for clothes. A muffin from Dunkin' Donuts costs 480 calories. Do you have enough calories to spend on a muffin? Eat what you need and what you can afford, not what you have to burn off later. Don't incur food debt.

Plan how and when you're going to exercise. Get out your calendar or PDA. What does the rest of your week look like? Do you go to an office every day? Do you have morning or afternoon appointments? Evening activities? If you plan your workouts around your obligations (also including your fun activities) and write them in your calendar, you won't have any excuse for not doing what you planned. Then use your PDA to find the closest well-stocked market and go there. Making life easy for yourself is what it's all about.

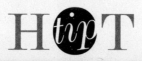

When you go to the supermarket, dress to look good! Not only is the market a great place to meet people, but also, if you look good, you'll feel good, and you'll buy food that's good for you. You don't have to wear six-inch platform stilettos; just no baggy sweats or anything that looks like you slept in it the night before. Clean skinny jeans or a neat pair of yoga pants and a fresh white tank or tee shirt can be totally hot and totally appropriate.

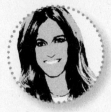

Kelly's Cardinal Rule

Give HOT! your all!

What's on your social calendar? Are you doing things you love? If not, you should be. If you do things that bore you, you won't have any reason to be HOT, and then you'll be boring to yourself and to others. If you think people aren't attracted or drawn to you, it's not because you aren't skinny; it's because you aren't *fun*.

Once you have a social plan it's time to make a clothing plan. What are you going to wear to each of the events you have coming up? Are the clothes clean, pressed, and in good repair? There's no bigger bummer than pulling a smokin' HOT outfit out of the closet and discovering there's a big stain in the front, or the hem is down, or there's a button missing. Sure, you could wear something else, but you probably won't feel as hot, and if you don't feel HOT you're not going to look your hottest either.

Finally, what's your hygiene and beauty plan? Do you need to schedule a haircut? Give yourself a manicure and pedicure? To feel good about yourself, you need to take care of yourself. That isn't selfish; it's what you deserve! Once you feel your hottest, you'll be able to give your best to your family and friends.

h⬤t button issue

I totally get what social networking is all about. I probably use it as much as anyone. But I don't confuse social networking with actually making connections with real humans—live and in person—people I love and enjoy. If you don't learn to manage your social networking online, or use it as a replacement for getting out in the world, it can ultimately take over (and even ruin) your life. The real world is a lot bigger, more exciting, and fun, so instead of getting lured into the virtual world, stay grounded in reality. We humans are naturally social animals; we enjoy being in a group dynamic. So turn off your hot new electronics and start to get HOT. Human contact is HOT; texting is not!

Tuesday: A Little *Ohm* and a Little Oh Yeah!—It's All About Balance

Today we're going to talk about exercise. I know, you hate that. But remember, you're reading this book because you want to know how to get HOT. I'm not going to lie to you; the fact is, I've never met a smokin' hot couch potato and I bet you haven't either. But don't worry; I'm not going to ask you to spend hours (or even one hour) in the gym every day for the rest of your life. For me, exercise is all about being energized, happy, and healthy; it isn't about being skinny. But if you're concerned about your weight, exercise will help you there, too. Exercise builds muscle, and muscle burns the calories that make up fat.

My own exercise routine (which I'll be sharing with you later on) combines aerobics and yoga, because life is all about balance. You can't be all movement without some stillness in your life, and you can't be all spiritual without a bit of fun. I'm sure even Gandhi cracked a smile from time to time.

If you work yourself to exhaustion first thing in the morning, you're defeating the purpose. I always say that your body is like a Ferrari, and exercising is like tuning up your engine so that it runs well for as long as you're on the go. My days are long—as I'm sure yours are, too. Exercise is what allows me to enjoy everything else I do in my life, whether it's writing, pursuing business opportunities, magazine editing, horseback riding, or raising my daughters. What do you love? Walking in the park? Skydiving? Gallery hopping? Those are forms of exercise, too! Moving *is* exercise.

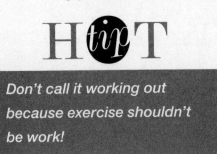

Don't call it working out because exercise shouldn't be work!

I'm not going to lie to you. I don't have all the time in the world to exercise. Sometimes I can only do twenty minutes, sometimes twenty-five, and sometimes I can do thirty minutes. But if you want to be HOT, you have to exercise every day. I truly believe that if you exercise intensely for twenty to thirty minutes on a daily basis, your heart will be healthy and you will both look and feel fit. If I told you that you needed to go to the gym for an hour a day, you probably wouldn't do it anyway, and truthfully, I probably wouldn't either. I believe in keeping it real! I also believe in challenging myself and bumping it up a notch one day a week. My favorite way to do that is to take a spin class, which is not only fun but also a great cardio workout.

I've been working with various coaches and trainers since I was eleven years old, and I've picked up many great tips along the way. My first swim coach told me to "always finish strong," and that's been my mantra ever since. One hundred percent is never mediocre. My former husband, who was in many ways my life coach, told me to complete at least one exercise routine once a day, and that's how I came up with my workout plans.

Unless you're training like a professional athlete, you probably don't need to eat very much, if at all, before you do your morning exercise. I do eat a couple of oranges in the morning and drink coffee. (I love coffee; I would probably marry coffee if it proposed.) Some studies have shown that caffeine helps to improve exercise performance and may also help you to burn more fat. On the other hand, it also restricts your blood vessels, which could be problematic. It's also a mild diuretic, so if you do drink coffee, you also need to drink water to keep yourself hydrated. As with most things, there are two sides to the argument. You really need to pay attention to what your body is telling you it needs.

My suggestion is to get up, do your exercise, shower, have something to eat, and start your day. The Centers for Disease

Control and Prevention Web site suggests that twenty minutes of moderate aerobic exercise each day can lower your risk for heart disease and stroke, two of the leading causes of death in the United States. If I can find twenty minutes in the morning to exercise, so can you!

Happy Twenty

I'm sure you've read that you need to exercise at least one hour a day, three times a week, but I'd rather keep my body moving for twenty minutes every day than stress it out on alternate days.

- Go for an easy 18-minute run.

- Pick up a dumbbell of whatever weight you can handle, hold it with both hands in front of you, and do 2 minutes of ballet squats, lowering your body until your thighs are parallel to the floor, then standing up straight and repeating the squat. (If you want to really feel hot, do your squats wearing high heels.)

Healthy Twenty-five

- Go for an easy 18-minute run.

- Jump rope for 2 minutes.

- Lie on your stomach with your legs stretched behind you and your hands slightly in front of your shoulders.

Tuck in your toes and lift your hips off the floor until your hands and legs are straight. Now stretch your body forward, bending your elbow until your body forms a straight line parallel to the floor. Return to your starting position and repeat. Do this for 2 minutes. In yoga this is called doing a Downward Dog to a Plank.

- Now turn on your back with your knees bent and feet flat on the floor. Keeping your shoulders flat on the floor, pressing down with your feet, raise your hips off the floor until you're making a straight line from knees to shoulders. In yoga, this is called a Bridge or a Backbend or a Half Wheel. Do this five times.

Hot Thirty

- Go for a 20-minute run.

- Do ballet squats for 3 minutes.

- Do the Downward Dog to a Plank for 3 minutes.

- Do 5 Bridges.

- With your back against the wall, squat so that your thighs are parallel to the ground and your butt is off the floor. Hold this position for 2 minutes. To help the time pass as you multiprocess, call your mom or a friend on your cell and complain about how much your legs are hurting!

H*tip*T

Run for your life! I know that if you're not a runner, the whole idea can make you tired before you've even begun. But there are ways to make it fun. Here are a few of my HOT tips for having a fun run:

- Make a "HOT pact" to run with a friend. Not only will you be more likely to do it if you've made a date, but also you can vent all your frustrations and tribulations about everything in your life while you're running. Get it all out and save the money you would have spent on therapy for a pair of hot new shoes. The secret is that if you're both running, your friend won't be able to hear half the things you're saying anyway; don't hold back.

- Run in the street instead of on the sidewalk. I took a lot of flack for this when they filmed me on Season 2 of the *Real Housewives of New York City*. The thing is, I think that people walking down the street while texting are a lot more dangerous than a car. Drivers will go out of their way to avoid you (accidents are too much paperwork, and they really mess up a day), but strolling texters will walk right into you without even seeing you. You could also get smacked by a shopping bag, a stroller, or even an oversized purse. Sidewalks are really obstacle courses. Beware!

- Watch out for bicycle messengers.

- Avoid smokers.

- Jump over potholes and count how many you have jumped.

- Wear clothing that isn't going to invite the kinds of comments you don't want to hear, such as "Come run my way!"

- Take money for a coffee at the end of your run.

- Never take a credit card on your run. Shop owners and other customers are offended by sweaty shoppers (and certainly sweaty people should not be trying on clothes).

H*tip*T

Kelly's Playlist

It's much more fun exercising to music. Here are a few tunes that will heat up your workout.

"Jolene" by Dolly Parton

"Sweet Disposition" by The Temper Trap

"Skinny Love" by Bon Iver

"Float On" by Modest Mouse

"Quelqu'un M'a Dit" by Carla Bruni

"Don't Stop Believing" by Journey

"I Hate that You Love Me" by Diddy

"Beautiful People" by Chris Brown

"Kids" by MGMT

"Move Like Jagger" by Maroon 5

So, Run for Your Life!

If you're feeling lethargic and dull, the best way I know to start feeling HOT is to get up and go. Now I run to make sure I have the energy and enthusiasm to participate fully in all aspects of my life. I never start my day without a twenty-minute run or a hug and a kiss from my girls. I could be on the beach, in the streets of Easthampton, New York, Paris, with or without a dog, but I run. I run for my life.

Get Leggier Legs

An April 10, 2009, article about me in *Harper's Bazaar* captioned one of the photos "She's got legs." I was born blessed with long, lean legs, but I work very hard to keep them looking the way they do. I'm tall, but I could just as easily have long, large legs. And long and large is not hot. Unfortunately I can't give you my legs. But I can help you to be the best *you* can be. Here are three exercises that will tone your legs so that even if they don't get longer, they'll look longer because they're leaner.

1. **BALLET SQUATS: Do 10 to 15 of these.**

2. **BRIDGE: Do 10 of these.**

3. **STORK: Stand (with your hand on the wall or the back of a chair if necessary for balance) and lift your right leg toward your chest. Hold that position for 30 seconds and repeat with your left leg. In yoga this is called the Stork pose. To make it more difficult you can also try doing a one-legged squat by bending the leg that's on the floor. Do 8 of these on each leg.**

How to Avoid the "Freshman Fifteen"

We've all heard about the dreaded fifteen pounds almost every college freshman seems to gain. But you don't have to. All you need to do is maintain a sense of balance and keep making good choices for yourself. Even if you're cooking for yourself, there are plenty of easy, healthy options. You don't need much equipment to make healthy meals for yourself, just one good knife, one nonstick frying pan, and one saucepan. Try my Extra-Easy Oatmeal (page 141) for breakfast; it doesn't even require any cooking. And even if all you have is a hot plate in a dorm room, you can still have Shrimp Taco Tuesdays (page 194), Bar No-Pitti Pasta (page 208), Bowties and Green Pearls (page 211), and Pineapple Fried Rice (page 218), to name just a few options, and, of course, any one of the many salad choices. Check out all the recipes and see which ones appeal to you—and I don't mean just the brownies or the cake!

Here are a few "Kelly rules" for keeping off that extra weight:

1. **Do 15 minutes of fun exercise every day:**

   - **Do 20 push-ups.**

   - **Do 20 sit-ups.**

   - **Do 20 jumping jacks.**

   - **Jump rope for 2 minutes.**

- Put on your headphones and dance it out until your time is up. Channel those dance parties you used to have in high school. Watch your moves in the mirror and have a party by yourself.

- Now sit on your bed, close your eyes, and think about what you're really good at. Get rid of any negative thoughts. Negative-town isn't Fun-town.

2. For every beer you drink, you owe me a glass of water.

3. For every piece of pizza, you owe me 20 sit-ups.

4. If you wake up hung over, you owe me a bottle of water and a 20-minute run.

5. For every cheeseburger and fries, you owe me 12 cartwheels on the quad with your friends.

6. For every milkshake, you owe me 50 jumping jacks.

7. If you starve yourself for a day because you want to lose weight for Homecoming, you owe me 5 minutes of sitting Indian style in a corner and meditating on why you thought that was a good option.

8. For every pint of ice cream you eat while studying or watching TV, you owe me a pint of nonfat yogurt instead (next time you have the craving).

H**tip**T

You are a living organism; life is an organic process. You need to be up and active, ready to enjoy the process. Be open and available and ready to do fun stuff. Participating in what you love is HOT.

You also need to become aware of what your particular body needs and how it responds to various types of exercise. If you're feeling a bit frazzled and you need to calm down, you might want to take a yoga class. Or if you're a bit down, you might need some Zumba to get the juices flowing. Some people do really well with weight training, but I've found that intensive weight training just makes me look big and muscular—not hot. Listen to your body and give it what it needs most.

Most of all I want you to try different things. When I was a competitive swimmer in my teens, I was swimming two to three hours every day, but I was also watching Jane Fonda's workout videos and moving along with her. I wanted to look like Jane Fonda, just like everyone else. I've also been riding horses since I was fifteen. Now, when I'm in the Hamptons, I ride every day. I love working with the horses, even if I do tend to treat them like my own pets. I carry "sweeties" and reward them for good behavior. People are always remarking on how much the horses love me, but that's because they don't know I have gooey peppermint sticking to my palms.

The point is not that I want you to do what I do, it's that I want you to be curious and adventurous. Do one thing every day that takes you out of your comfort zone. When Bravo approached me to join the cast of the *Real Housewives of New York City*, I'd never done reality TV. It was a huge leap of faith for me, and while it wasn't always fun and games (to put it mildly),

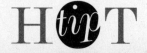

Don't be afraid to drink water while working out. Keep the intensity, but hydrate when you can.

I have absolutely no regrets. While I don't expect you to show up on reality television, I do want you to take chances. Do something new even if it's something relatively small. Pop in an exercise video and dance along—no one is watching. Try tap dancing. Go rollerblading. Take a new route to work; try a fruit you've never eaten; say hi to someone you've never said hi to before. Don't be afraid to look foolish. There's nothing more foolish than sitting on your butt when you could be moving your body and having fun.

hot button issue

People who complain about things they *can* change make me crazy. Instead of complaining, get on the treadmill and work it out. Or, in the words of Dr. Phil, "If you don't like it, change it."

Wednesday:
Diet =
"DIE with a T"

I don't believe in diets; diets are for people who want to get skinny. I want you to be happy. If you feel good about yourself, you'll make good choices. If you starve yourself to be skinny, you'll be undermining your sense of self-worth and you'll be unhappy every day. Eating well—a variety of high-quality, fresh, unprocessed foods—is for people who want to be happy—and if you're not happy you won't be hot!

Happy is always better than skinny. We always hear people saying things like, "Oh, when I lose ten pounds I'll meet the right guy," but losing ten pounds isn't going to help you meet Mr. Right; a good self-image will.

It seems to me that most women fall into one of two categories. The first is the overachiever who tries hard, exercises, wants to be her best, look her best, and have the best. The second is the underachiever who thinks she'll never be good enough, who waits instead of acts, then blames and shames the world for not being there for her. I want you to aspire to be an overachiever who always tries to be her best. "Try" is the operative word.

Here's how to do that:

- **Make good choices.**

- **Be vain; vanity is actually about self-preservation.**

- **Take care of yourself and your friends.**

- **When in doubt, have fun.**

- **When you're sad, cry to a friend, not to a bucket of KFC.**

- **When you're down on yourself, ask anyone anywhere "How are *you*?"**

- **Keep smiling.**

Stay positive and move forward. This is your last try at today. Yesterday may not have been great, but, today is better—you just need to see it that way. The choice is up to you.

I've already said that you need to treat your body like a Ferrari, but maybe you prefer a Maserati, an Aston Martin, a Corvette, or even a Bentley. Whatever your luxury car of choice, if you treat it well, it will increase in value; if you treat it like a bargain rental car, it's just going to wear out—and being worn out is not hot! I assume you wouldn't fill up your luxury car with cheap, sub-optimal gas. So why would you try to fuel your body with poor-quality food? Or try to run it on empty? Eating well is 80 percent of maintaining a healthy weight. Exercise is keeping the engine moving. Don't confuse the two. It's not about working out more so that you can eat whatever you want. If you're not nourishing yourself well, no matter how much you exercise, you won't be getting the most out of what you're doing. As a young athlete I'd always known that, but when I started modeling and listening to everyone telling me I needed to lose ten pounds, everything I'd known flew out the window. I lost my way and had to get back on the right track.

When we were both nineteen and living in Paris, model Elaine Irwin and I tried the white diet. For several days we ate nothing but cereal and rice. It certainly gave us a lot of energy, but it was also boring. It wasn't any fun sitting at a café with our friends wearing our tight black miniskirts (the model's uniform of the '90s) and watching them enjoy their dinner while we ate nothing because we'd already consumed enough rice and cereal for an entire small nation. After a few days we were both starving and bored.

What did I learn from that? Food deprivation does two things: It makes you irritable and it leads to binge eating.

HtipT

Model diet secrets that DON'T work. (I've even tried some myself!)

- Eating nothing but cereal and rice for days does *not* work.

- Cigarettes do *not* work.

- Drugs do *not* work.

- The alcohol diet does *not* work.

- Binging and purging does *not* work. In fact, it makes your face look bloated. Who wants a thin body and a fat face!

- Diuretic teas do *not* work.

- Enemas do *not* work.

- The Graham cracker diet does *not* work.

When it comes to food choices, I've probably made every mistake in the book. A real biggie occurred when I was about to give birth to my daughter Sea. I remember it clearly to this day. I was sitting on the red leather couch in our apartment and I felt my first contraction. I immediately screamed to my husband, who, having gone through it before,

- A vegetarian diet with no starch and no protein does *not* work.

- The tapeworm diet does *not* work. Instead of making you thin, it makes you dead.

- Eating nothing but an apple a day for a week does *not* work (although it does save you money).

- Liquid diets do *not* work. They don't teach you how to eat well; they just teach you how to *not* eat.

- Eating Kleenex to make yourself feel full does *not* work.

- Strict diets of any kind do *not* work. (Rules are meant to be broken.)

- Starving yourself does *not* work.

went to the gym. I'd been told that you should eat light when you're about to give birth, so I decided I needed to eat and ordered Chinese chicken soup with noodles. But what I got was more like chicken with vegetables and rice—swimming in tons of brown sauce. Back from the gym, Gilles watched me eat the entire thing. Hours later, he watched me throw it all up, and took me to the hospital where I was put on an IV drip because I was dehydrated. The moral of this story is that you can't eat whatever you want at any time, even though you want it. You just can't; sorry to disappoint. I'd overloaded my already overloaded body and it rebelled. The second time is always a charm and I knew what to expect. So before giving birth to my second daughter, Teddy, I had a turkey sandwich and she came flying out before the doctor had even arrived.

I've been on crash diets; I've been on juice fasts; I've tried to get through the day eating nothing more than an apple. I can tell you from personal experience that none of those options are healthy—and they don't work. Now my best way to detox is just to avoid eating any unhealthy foods for a few days.

I'm stubborn—I admit it. If someone tells me no, I have to try it. Everyone had been telling me that I wasn't the juicing type and I would hate it. Well, they were right. When I started the juice fast, Season 2 of the *Real Housewives of New York City* was airing and the ladies' strategy was to team up against me. I don't like confrontational women; I like team players. When I was accused of being a "bitch" on national television, I was really upset. My response was to find comfort in Mexican food and margaritas for lunch and dinner three days straight. When I realized my "Mexican fiesta" was unhealthy and was not solving any problems, I decided to juice on a liquid diet from Liquiteria in NYC. Basically, greens, carrots, and beet juice is the concept. The reality for me was no chewing, no caffeine, and headaches (!) for three more days, which was almost torture for me. It's not that I'm against juicing; I

THE KELLY GREEN DIET

This is how I get back on track after I've overindulged. I do a minicleanse, which I call the Kelly Green Diet. I have:

- **2 green juices in the morning (see recipe on page 247)**

- **a KKBfit lunch including protein, vegetables, and carbs with 1 green juice**

- **a KKBfit dinner including protein and vegetables**

Between meals I drink only water with lemon juice to help flush out my system. It works for me. Just because you overeat at one meal (or more) doesn't mean you have to punish your body. Don't scold it; nurture it.

actually love green juices. It's just that I don't believe in using juices as substitutes for food. The human body is not meant to run on liquids alone. For me it's all about balance, and to keep my body in balance, I need to *eat* real food. When I don't eat, my body doesn't operate well, and I don't like the way I feel. That doesn't mean I wouldn't have a green juice after a run, but I've learned—by making the mistake—that I don't function well without real food in my diet.

On the last day of my juice fast, I took my older daughter to a Yankees game where we gorged on sushi. (Yes, they have sushi at Yankee Stadium.) As a result, I was stuffed and blinded by carbs when A-Rod came up to bat and hit a home run. Was I able to savor that A-Rod moment with my daughter? Absolutely not. I was in a food coma. Will I ever let myself be thrown into a Mexican food frenzy again? No! Lesson learned: I made another stupid food choice, and because of that choice I missed that home run moment with my daughter. From now on, when I go to a Yankees game I'll have a small hot dog instead. . . . I want you to do the same: Be present, so that you don't miss a moment of whatever life throws your way.

When you're HOT, food is not your enemy. When you know what's going to fuel your day, you can stop obsessing about your carrot intake and concentrate on what it is that's going to make you a great person in life and enable you to do the things you love. I care more about your life plan than your meal plan. Did you go to the beach this summer? Do you hang out with your friends? Have you put on some great music or danced to your own tune?

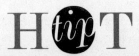

Lonely breeds loneliness. Get out there and make it a point to be around people you like who like the people you like and the activities you like. Toxic friends and toxic activities are not hot.

I like to think of my life plan as a "Kelly pie." Food is just one small wedge of the pie. The rest of the pie is made up of family, friends, fun, work, sleep, and charity, which means doing something for another person without being asked and without being compensated. If food is all you think about, you're missing out on the rest of your life. I don't want you to spend your life thinking about food.

My ideal twenty-four-hour life-plan:

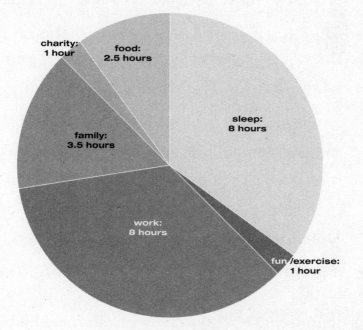

How would you divide up your own pie? Following are some hints to help you get started:

1. Celebrate your own health. We take health for granted.

2. Get up in the morning and say, "I'm so grateful to be where I am and look the way I do," no matter what your size is.

3. Tell yourself you look HOT, because you do.

4. Believe in your ability to make good choices today and every day.

5. Be mindful of what you eat. If I have to be mindful of what I eat, so do you. We're in this together.

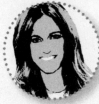

Kelly's Cardinal Rule

You can't outsmart your metabolism, but you can jump-start it by eating nutritious, well-rounded meals. If you don't eat enough, your body will think it's starving and your metabolism will automatically slow down to preserve as much energy and body fat as possible. If you feed your body what it needs, your metabolism will work for you instead of against you.

Is this you? *I don't eat breakfast; I eat chicken and lettuce for lunch; and I eat a salad with vegetables and light dressing at night.* If that's you, you are trying to be skinny, but actually you're not ever going to trim down. You're starving your body, even though you think you "eat nothing" . . . and are on a "skinny track."

Write down what you ate for the last two days. Don't lie. We can start fresh tomorrow, one bite at a time.

What I Eat Every Day

To begin with, I'm not a big breakfast person. My three go-to breakfasts are either two oranges or a plate of mixed berries if I'm not going to be very active; all-bran cereal or some other high-fiber cereal with almond milk or unsweetened coconut milk if I'm going on a long run, riding, or doing something else that requires extra energy; and on weekends, I love making pancakes to eat with my girls. We make them with coconut milk and top them with fresh fruit. You don't always need syrup; low-glycemic-index agave nectar is delicious, too. Sometimes I even go against Miss Manners and eat them with my hands. (My Favorite Pancakes, page 142).

Every morning is different. Some days I'll wake up and have the time and the energy to make pancakes. Other mornings a green drink (Kelly Green Juice, page 247) or a smoothie may be all you can tackle. My kids and I love smoothies, and I make them all the time as an easy breakfast alternative. The point is that no child or adult should ever leave the house in the morning without something in their stomachs. A plastic cup that says "Forced Family Fun" from www.themonogramshops.com makes the smoothie go down with a giggle.

HOT tip

People try to control their meal plan when they can't control other things in their life. That's how eating disorders are born. Stop micromanaging your meals and take control of your whole life.

hot button issue

People often ask me how I feel about snacks. Do I snack? What are my go-to snack choices? My answer is that I truly believe that if you eat three good meals a day you shouldn't really need to snack between meals. I was married to a Frenchman, and the French philosophy is not to snack. But sometimes, I do sneak a snack here and there. If you really feel the need to snack, please do, but first *stop* and ask yourself if you're really hungry. Don't eat because you're bored, and certainly don't snack to keep your mouth busy while your eyes are glued to the television. If you're bored, get out and do something. Sitting alone in front of the TV eating ice cream is *not hot*! Food is energy; it shouldn't be mistaken for comfort or entertainment, or a friend/enemy.

I know that eating a pint of ice cream can make you feel really good—for the moment. But what are the ramifications? How much more will you have to exercise to work off those calories? Is the momentary gratification really worth the long-term results? How much extra weight do you really want to carry around every day? Personally I don't ever want to carry anything heavier than my own purse.

Try to make at least one day a week a "no-snack day." I promise that it won't be as difficult as you might think.

Lunch is my biggest meal, because I need the energy to get me through my busy days. I might have brown rice with vegetables and a protein such as chicken, tofu, or fish. I call this "Energy Economics": eating what my body needs based on the action of the day. When I'm really busy and active, I can't eat as if I were at a spa. Spa food is great when I'm relaxing, but I don't live at a spa, and neither do you, so you will need more food to keep you going.

In the evening, your body needs less energy, so you need less food. For dinner, I eat something light, like a salad and a protein or soup and a salad. I've actually been eating soup and salad for dinner since I was a little girl. When I was young, my parents used to pack the entire family—my twin brother, my sister, and I—into the car and take road trips from our home in Illinois to Montreal, Aspen, and even as far as Washington, D.C. My

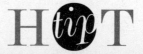

A great way to combine your meat and vegetables is by stuffing. Stuff cabbage, sweet peppers, tomatoes, or even onions with ground meat, chicken, or turkey seasoned with salt and pepper. Bake until the meat is cooked through and the vegetable is softened. If you mix the ground meat with cooked rice, you've got a whole meal in one neat package. See Have an Impromptu Pepper Party (page 224).

mother loved going to the best restaurants and hotels in the country, but we were a party of five, and that sometimes got expensive. Whichever restaurant we went to, my parents ordered soup and salad for us kids. It was inexpensive, came to the table quickly, and allowed me to nap on some of the finest linens made in America. That's the truth; I grew up on soup and salad.

When I was in my twenties, modeling and traveling the world, I learned how to make healthy, inexpensive, easy dinners out of a can. Many people think that models lead super glamorous lives filled with jet-set vacations and nightclub outings. That's a total misconception. Whether I was in Paris or Africa, it was usually just for a few days, and usually I was working with people I didn't know. I figured out that all I needed was a can of peas, a can of stewed tomatoes, and a hotplate, and I could have a meal ready in no time. I called it Kelly Green Peezzz. Even now, when I need a quick, healthy dinner, I still revert to my twenties and make that, only now I dress it up with truffle salt, garlic powder, and crushed red pepper flakes.

Since I try to work out in the mornings, I stay away from starchy carbs in the evening because I know I don't need the quick energy and I won't be actively burning them off. If I've had a substantial lunch, I don't need to eat a big dinner.

If I don't eat that way, I'm violating my own laws of energy economics and my body goes either into inflation mode (too much energy when I don't need it) or recession mode (not enough energy in the bank for me to draw from). The key is to create economic equilibrium: eating well so that I feel good, which allows me to be happy.

To summarize:

FOR SIX DAYS

- **Fruit or a cup of cereal with milk in the morning.**

- **A substantial lunch including 1 cup of carbs with a protein.**

- **Protein with salad or vegetables for dinner.**

ON THE SEVENTH DAY

- **Have fun and indulge yourself.**

Of course, I can't eat perfectly every single day, and I don't expect you to be perfect, either. None of us live in a test-tube, and life happens. Maybe you have a business dinner one night, or you get stuck in traffic, or you're really backed up with work. When something happens to throw you off course, just be sure you get back on track the next day—no excuses!

Kelly's Cardinal Rule

Eat to live well, not to survive.

Finally, I try not to eat after eight o'clock at night unless it's for my work. I do try to eat with my girls as often as I can before I go out. I'm not in fourth grade and I can't say that I eat at 6:30 p.m. every night, but if you invite me to a late dinner, you would have to be the funniest person on the planet for me to accept!

When I break my own rules, I get into trouble—a lesson I learned the hard way. In 1996, I had one week before going to St. Bart's to do a photo shoot for *Elle* magazine, and Gilles, my husband at the time, would be the photographer. One of my friends had gone on a no-carb diet for five days and lost weight, so I decided to try it. How bad could it be? I worked out every day as usual and didn't eat any carbs the entire time. My face looked visibly thinner, but by the fourth day I felt weak. On the sixth day, as we boarded the flight at 6:00 a.m. for St. Maarten, where we would change planes for St. Bart's, I was exhausted. I took a bag of Snyder's of Hanover pretzels (my five days of no carbs were over) with me in case I got hungry, but I didn't really recognize my own hunger anymore; I just felt tired. We flew all day and when we landed it was hot. I ate a little fish that night and went to bed early because my head was pounding. The next day when I was getting my hair and makeup done, I felt faint. I had absolutely no energy, my smile was upside down, and I was very quiet. Gilles, who usually couldn't get me to stop talking, realized that something was wrong. His nickname for me is Kiki, and I overheard him remarking to the stylist, "Kiki isn't being Kiki." As soon as we'd completed the first shot, in a graveyard, no less, my husband threw me in the water to cool down and to make me laugh again. No carbs is *no bueno*! Lesson learned.

We all have occasions when we want to lose a few pounds quickly. We just need to do it the right way. Here's what I keep in mind today: A *Real* Supermodel Diet nurtures and restores, it *doesn't* deprive. That's the philosophy for The KKB 3-Day Supermodel diet:

THE KKB 3-DAY SUPERMODEL DIET

- Cut out oils, alcohol (in a glass and in your food), sugar, nuts, salt, and caffeine—no cheating.

- For breakfast have 2 oranges or Kelly Green Juice (page 247).

- For lunch have brown rice or a grain without sauce, chicken, and vegetables.

- For dinner have steak, chicken, or shrimp with steamed spinach and a squeeze of lemon juice.

- Drink a glass of water with lemon juice after dinner.

- Switch your plates: Make your dinner plate your salad plate and vice versa for portion control.

- Chew your food 8 times instead of 3 or 4.

- Brush your teeth and chew mint gum as soon as you finish eating. When your mouth is fresh and minty you'll be less tempted to eat again.

- Drink 8 to 10 glasses of water a day—any more can cause water intoxication.

- Take a multivitamin every day.

- Do 20 minutes of light, restorative exercise—biking, walking, yoga, Pilates—every day.

- Sleep 8 hours every night.

- Nurture yourself: have a mani-pedi, take a bath, use a body scrub and baby oil, blow out your hair, put on eyeliner and mascara, and blush your checks.

Meet Kelly's Food Plate

I'm sure you've heard all about the food pyramid (now morphed into the food plate) that the USDA created in order to guide us toward a healthier diet. I strongly urge you to eat everything on your plate so that you don't wind up eating off someone else's plate later on.

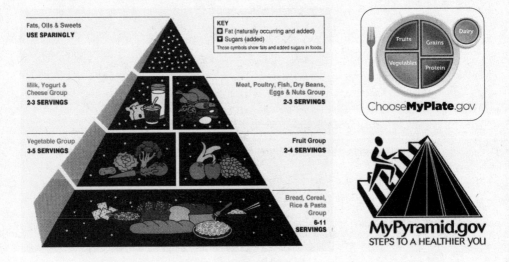

It's interesting to me that the USDA's recommendations have evolved over time. My own food plate has also evolved over time, mainly through trial and error. Every time I've tried cutting out carbs and eating more fat, my body has rebelled. When I skip meals, I don't have the energy I need to do what I want or what I need to do. What I'm sharing with you is what has worked for me. I want you to eat enough food so that you have the right energy to function at the top of your game.

My own personal food image, although based on My Plate, is like a pear-shaped diamond—smallest at the tip (my breakfast), wide in the middle (a nutritious, filling lunch), and smaller at the bottom (a light meal in the evening). This is one instance when, in my opinion, a diamond really is a girl's best friend. But, guys, if you're buying me a diamond, make it round.

According to WebMD, adult women need about 46 grams of protein and men need about 55 grams a day. I eat meals that include a lot of protein not just because I crave it but because I know that we need protein to build muscle, and muscle burns more calories than fat even when your body is at rest. WebMD reports that, according to Christopher Wharton, Ph.D., a certified personal trainer and researcher with the Rudd Center for Food Policy and Obesity at Yale University, "10 pounds of muscle would burn 50 calories in a day spent at rest, while 10 pounds of fat would burn 20 calories." Protein also keeps us feeling full—longer than carbs or fat—and slows down the metabolism of carbohydrates so that our blood sugar doesn't spike and then drop. It's those blood sugar spikes that leave us feeling sleepy and heavy, and send us looking for something sugary to get us going again. We also need fat to make tissue and create certain biochemicals such as hormones, and we need carbohydrates for quick energy.

hot button issue

Just because I don't eat chocolate bars doesn't mean I can't eat candy. I *love* candy—particularly jelly beans. You might even say that I'm obsessed with jelly beans. If you're a fan of the *Real Housewives of New York City* you probably remember that on Season 3 I took a lot of flack for eating jelly beans and talking about processed and unprocessed foods. I was actually making light of that food snob moment. Who stops at a gas station and asks for carrots? Did you bring your organic food cooler with you on this road trip? The important point is not to be a food snob; but when in doubt choose the best option. Sometimes it's better to be happy than it is to be right. Was I able to make my point? Clearly it wasn't in the cards at that moment. Nevertheless, if you eat well the majority of the time, a handful of jelly beans isn't going to kill you.

I'm not sure where my candy obsession originated. It may have been because my childhood swim coach used to give us all about a tablespoon of Jell-O powder before a meet to give us a quick energy boost. Or it may have been because I used to hide my Halloween candy under the bed so that my brother and sister wouldn't steal it.

To this day, jelly beans, Jolly Ranchers, and red Twizzlers are still my absolute favorite treats for a sweet pick-me-up. I truly believe that everyone should enjoy a little sugar for a sweeter life.

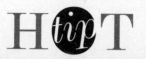

H tip T

Be curious! When you go to the supermarket, take a look around. If you see something you love, think of what you could do with it that you've never done before. Strawberries? Watermelon? Throw them in a salad. My daughters are both very adventurous eaters, and they've inspired me to be more adventurous myself. They eat quiche, bean salads, sushi . . . things I would never have eaten at their age.

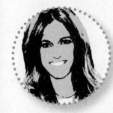

Kelly's Cardinal Rule

Whatever else you eat, you *must* eat a vegetable at lunch and dinner.

Although there are some things I choose not to eat— such as chocolate bars—I don't believe that any food should be forbidden, because the thing that is forbidden is sure to become the thing you want most. As I've said, I'm stubborn. When I was sixteen years old and the Elite Modeling Agency told me that I needed to lose ten pounds, the first thing I did was call a close friend who was living in New York. We walked around the city as I ate a DoveBar while telling him about the weight I "needed" to lose. Nowadays, I don't turn to chocolate as a comfort food when I'm stressed. I eat a lot of fruit, particularly in the morning because it gets me going without weighing me down. I like to mix different kinds of berries because they look so colorful and appetizing in a bowl, over cereal or yogurt.

Color is important for a variety of reasons. Having different colors on your plate makes the meal more appealing, but those different colored foods also provide different nutrients. There's absolutely no reason why you, wherever you live, can't eat "colorful" foods. All over the country there are "gi-normous" supermarkets where fruit and vegetable aisles are bursting with every color of the rainbow. The days when all you could get in Dayton (no offense to Dayton intended) was iceberg lettuce and pale pink tomatoes are long gone! In fact, I love going to the supermarket in every city I visit. The variety of foods I find is just amazing.

In February 2011, I was invited by Generosity Water (www.generositywater.org) to go to Haiti. I'd raised money to help them bring clean water to the country and they asked me to go and see one of the wells I'd helped to build. When I got there, I was first taken aback to see so many kids eating mainly pasta and hot dogs for lunch, but then I realized that they really didn't have any other options. They ate what was available to them to get the energy they needed. Generosity Water's purpose in providing clean water is to make it possible for the Haitian people to farm and, therefore, eat more fresh vegetables. At the same time, clean water improves sanitation, which will lead to better health.

Luckily, most of us in America have all these things; we just need to make healthier choices among all the options that are available to us.

That's the good news. The bad news is that abundance

can be confusing—not to mention tempting. Like department stores with displays of gorgeous options, food markets are also designed to get you to buy. All that colorful, fun packaging can make the food appear as enticing as a pair of Manolo Blahniks. You can go to a market with a list and the best of intentions . . . and then it happens. You're mesmerized by the unlimited possibilities, and you want it all. It's happened to me, so I know what it's like. If you go to a market such as Whole Foods, all the exotic ingredients from far-off lands are enough to send your taste buds on a world tour. I think it's great to try new things and figure out how you can mix and match what's there to make a FrenAsian or an ItaloGreek meal. But if you're not careful, you can also come home with over-loaded shopping bags and an empty wallet. So, when you go to a food store, approach it like a department store: Be conscious of the distractions, and don't get carried away by the temptations.

Here are a few tips on how to avoid the pits those sneaky food marketers are hoping you'll fall into when you enter their stores:

1. **Always go with a list and never buy more than two items you planned on taking home.**

2. **Bakery items are most often right at the front of the store so that you'll be more likely to load them in your cart right away, when you're not too tired, out of money, or out of time after walking up and down the aisles.**

3. **Staples like eggs, butter, and milk are often at the**

back of the store so that you have to walk through tempting aisles of junk food to get to them. Instead of walking through the center of the market, walk around the perimeter where all the fresh produce is displayed (and avoid the freezers full of ice cream).

4. If the supermarket has a pharmacy, it's probably there to tempt you to shop while your prescription is being filled. Phone your prescription in ahead of time so that it will be ready when you arrive to pick it up.

5. Be careful about stocking up on sale items. Very often they are products reaching their sell-by date that the market wants you to buy before they have to remove them from the shelves. Whenever you're buying an item with a sell-by date, check the ones in the back to see if the date is farther in the future than the ones in the front. When markets restock the shelves, they often move the older items to the front to sell first— and the same is true of fresh produce. Take it from the back where it's likely to be fresher.

6. Waiting to check out can be dangerous. Tempting goodies are often kept at or near the cash registers where you're likely to pick them up on impulse. If you can, try to shop "off hours" when the lines will be shorter.

7. *Don't* go food shopping when you're hungry! Not only will you want to eat everything in sight, but also, if your blood sugar is low your judgment may be impaired— just like when you've had too much alcohol to drink.

Foods to avoid:

- Most commercial cereals—they have enough sugar to be packaged candy

- Most soups—they're packed with sodium

- Packaged breads and rolls—except for pitas

- Chips—except for kale chips or baked pita chips

Here's a list of brand name and generic market foods I like to buy:

Annie's Boxed Mac & Cheese

Bumble Bee water-packed tuna

Goya canned black beans (for beans and rice)

Cerignola olives

Ginger beer

Land O'Lakes unsalted butter

Luigi Italian Ices: chocolate and lemon

Odwalla Superfood smoothies

Organic popcorn with no salt or oil

Skinny Cow ice cream desserts

Sriracha hot sauce

Stonyfield low-fat yogurt

Sun-dried tomatoes

Vita Coco Coconut Water

Whole wheat Italian Taralli Pugliesi (good replacement to croutons)

Even though supermarkets have a great variety of really healthy foods, there are some items I still tend to buy at Whole Foods or other large specialty markets. Here's what's often on my list.

Agave

Almond butter

Annie Chung's sauces

Arugula

Avocados

Bananas

Blueberries

Broccoli

Brussels sprouts

Cabbage

Celery

Cornmeal

Dark breads rich in grains

Dates

Dog treats

Eggs

Feta cheese

Freshly grated Parmesan cheese

Honey

Jalapeño salt

Lavender pepper

Mesclun salad

Mushrooms

Olive oil

Pita bread

Plain hummus (can be "dressed" up with jalapeños, red peppers, tomatoes, pepper, lemon)

Plum tomatoes

Raspberries

Red peppers

Serrano peppers

Shallots

Shitake/oyster mushroom combination packs

Sliced marcona almonds

Sliced beets

Soy milk (Soy nog for the Holidays!)

Spinach

Sugar snap peas

Sweet potatoes

Vanilla sugar

Whole-wheat couscous

Yams

H*tip*T

We should all try to buy the healthiest food we can find and afford. "Try" is the operative word here. If possible, I'd love you to buy organic, but I know how expensive that can be. I recently walked out of an organic market having paid $400 for just three bags of groceries. If you can't buy organic, buy something that's natural and fresh; if you can't buy fresh, buy frozen or even canned. In fact, in the winter when good tomatoes are hard to find, you'll get much better flavor if you cook with Italian canned plum tomatoes.

"Organic," in any case, seems like something of a misnomer to me. I know the Food and Drug Administration has regulations for certifying foods organic, but to me, for foods to be truly and totally organic, they would have to be grown in a test tube or a greenhouse with no exposure to the natural elements. We're all exposed to impurities every day, and so are any foods grown or raised in a natural environment. According to Charles Stuart Platkin, Ph.D., M.P.H., whose syndicated health, nutrition, and fitness column, "The Diet Detective," appears in more than 100 daily newspapers, "When organic vegetables are grown in the midst of conventional crops, pesticide drift is hard to prevent. Low levels of pesticides can remain in the soil thirty years after the product was applied, and sometimes pesticides in irrigation water lead to detectable levels in an organic field." So please don't get unnecessarily hung up on buying organic.

Just be sure to read the label and buy the best you can find. Become a comparison food shopper. Avoid heavy syrups, added sugar, and foods loaded with sodium. There are many frozen and canned foods that don't have all these unnecessary added ingredients. And don't buy foods whose labels are full of words you can't pronounce. If you can't pronounce it and you don't know where it came from, it probably isn't good for you.

What I really want you to do is eat as healthfully as you can in the environment you're in.

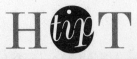

We eat with our eyes—creating a palette—as well as our palates. A white palette may look great in the bathroom but not on a dinner plate. I think of each meal as a way to "color me beautiful." Bright red strawberries, purplish blueberries, orange carrots or yams, gorgeous ripe tomatoes, dark green broccoli, spinach, or other greens all have different kinds of antioxidants, which are chemicals found only in plants and help to slow down the process of internal aging. The younger we are on the inside, the hotter we'll feel and look on the outside.

I also believe that *how* you eat is as important as *what* you eat. Eating ought to be a total experience; it isn't just about stuffing food in your mouth to fill yourself up. It's also about taking time for quiet reflection or for conversation and laughing with family and friends. Let's face it. You're not starving. You're not worrying where your next meal is coming from. No one's going to swoop down and snatch the food off your plate if you don't eat it fast enough—so turn off your cell phone and engage in conversation.

I've seen how Europeans eat as a matter of course. They put their knives and forks down between bites and talk. They set the table with a cloth or placemats, nice china, and cutlery. They drink from glasses, not a bottle, can, or a paper cup. And they don't put paper cartons, bottles, or jars on the dining table. "Dining" is the operative word here. Try it. You can even splurge and use cloth napkins.

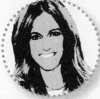

Kelly's Cardinal Rule

Plate your food as if it were being served to you in a fine restaurant. Use a fancy foreign accent as you invite everyone to come to the table. Or try saying it in French. My girls love it when I announce, *"Le dîner est servi!"*

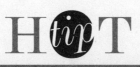

Fast food doesn't have to be fat food. Tomato and scrambled eggs is fast but not fat. A slice of commercial pizza is both fast and fat. Sprinkling sugar and cinnamon on your popcorn is fast; eating the entire bowl is fat. When I was a teenager, I'd go to a fast food place and order large fries—not a good choice. Not so long ago, I made another bad choice. I was looking for something that would be "fast," and I came up with ramen noodles. Not a good idea. I didn't think I was eating very much but I actually seemed to be gaining weight. I finally figured out that I was retaining tons of water from all the sodium in the noodles. It wasn't the noodles themselves—if I'd been eating pasta or brown rice I would have been fine—it was all that salt! There are always fast options that won't make you fat. It's just up to you to choose them.

Some Fast (Not Fat) Go-To Foods

- Steamed broccoli: My kids were raised on broccoli and organic pasta. This is my diet when I'm filming or have to be photographed.

- Oranges: I eat 2 every morning.

- Steamed spinach: My daughter Teddy's favorite side for eggs.

- Blueberries: My after-exercise snack.

- Turkey: My go-to sandwich on whole wheat bread (try cracked pepper turkey).

- Soy: If you see me in Starbucks, I am ordering a Venti Iced Soy Chai Latte (with an extra shot of espresso when necessary).

- Yogurt, 2% fat (I don't feed my girls food that's had all the fat removed, and I don't eat it, either. It usually means they've added something else we shouldn't be eating—or else it doesn't taste good.)

- Salmon: I love baked salmon. It is a surprisingly easy dinner to make. (See Easy Baked Salmon with Fennel, page 200)

- Nuts (especially almonds): A must for every salad.

- Beans (and rice): My go-to high-energy meal.

- Tomatoes

Even when I'm eating at home alone with my girls, we are mindful of the total dining experience. At first you'll have to think about it. Make yourself pause between bites. Pay attention to the conversation around you. Soon enough you'll find that these good habits become automatic. Mindful dining is totally different from mindless eating. Mindless eating is sitting in front of the television with a bag of potato chips or walking down the street slurping on an ice cream cone. You're not really aware of how many chips you're consuming and you're probably rushing to finish that cone before it starts to melt and run down your arm. So how much can you really be enjoying what you're eating? How much are you really taking in of the program you're watching or your surroundings on the street?

Another one of my rules is to never skip a meal. You need to keep your internal engine running smoothly and it can't do that when it's running on the fumes at the bottom of the tank. Skipping meals won't make you hot. It also won't make you skinny because you'll be so starving that you'll probably eat more than you need at your next meal. Here's what they call people who skip meals: exhausted, irritable, and grumpy. If I don't eat three meals a day, I am really grumpy—like get-me-my-broomstick grumpy. I work out every day, so I need to fuel my engine. Bad food choices affect my life choices.

Now that you know what I eat, and how I believe you should be eating in order to look and feel HOT, I also want you to know that, as you'll soon see, Sunday is the day when all bets are off and you can eat whatever you please—within reason. Sunday is Funday, a day of indulgence.

hot button issue

One question people frequently ask me is whether I believe in taking vitamins or supplements, and the answer is "yes, I do," because, even though I know my diet is healthy, I can't be sure that I'm getting all the nutrients I need. All the vitamins and minerals we need can be found naturally in foods, but how do we know, even if we're eating a healthy diet, that we're getting everything we need? I don't want to take that chance. I think of the food I eat as my fuel and vitamins as my oil—my body's engine needs both. Vitamins and supplements are not food replacements, but we're exposed to so many environmental toxins on a daily basis that I believe we need to supplement our diets to counteract all the harm those substances can cause.

I take a prenatal multivitamin daily (I am not, nor am I expecting to become pregnant any time soon, but you never know . . .) because prenatal vitamins contain iron, calcium, and folic acid, as well as other B vitamins. Folic acid not only protects against birth defects; it also helps to promote heart health and prevent cell changes that could lead to cancer. In addition, I find that these vitamins give me more energy, are great for my nails and hair, and get rid of the dark circles under my eyes. Honestly, if I don't take them, I can see the difference.

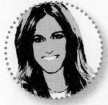

Kelly's Cardinal Rule

Never eat while you're doing something else, except enjoying good conversation. (And don't smack your *lips*, no matter how good the food tastes.) When you do two things at once, you're not doing either one of them properly. If you believe the food you eat while you're walking doesn't have any calories, you're wrong!

Thursday:
Tricks of My Trade

Now that you've got the basics, I'm going to share some of the tricks I use to kick-start my energy when I'm not feeling too hot, and some of the mistakes I've made along the way, so that you can learn from what I've learned. I'm actually glad for the mistakes I've made because anyone who doesn't make mistakes doesn't learn, and if you don't learn, you're boring! I'm sure you'll still be making some mistakes of your own, but you might as well learn what you can from mine instead of repeating them.

One of my biggest lessons came when I was competing in my very first horse show in Sagaponack, New York. I knew that I'd be jumping three rounds of eight 2-foot, 6-inch jumps set in three different courses. I knew I'd need lots of energy and decided to have a filling and nutritious lunch of pasta, broccoli, and shrimp. All great, but the show was running late and by four o'clock in the afternoon my adrenaline was pumped high and to me it felt as if I were starving. I decided to have an egg on a bagel from the food-service van. That turned out to be not so great. I was hot and sweaty and feeling like a stuffed Thanksgiving turkey. I wasn't energized. I was totally lethargic. I did all right in the competition, but I wasn't relaxed and I was pushing and pulling my horse instead of letting him go.

What lesson did I learn from that unhappy experience? To never eat more than I normally would, especially when I need to be physically active. In this case, my adrenaline was pumping but my blood sugar wasn't dropping.

What could I have done differently? I should have hydrated more when I started to feel hungry. On a recent Thanksgiving when I was fox hunting in North Carolina, it almost happened to me again. But this time I had granola with soy milk and a banana, and I drank a couple of bottles of water and a cup of coffee, so I could gallop through the hills. Even though I was anxious, I was hydrated, and I had a great time. Anxiety doesn't mean you're hungry; it means you're anxious. Food doesn't help anxiety and neither does alcohol.

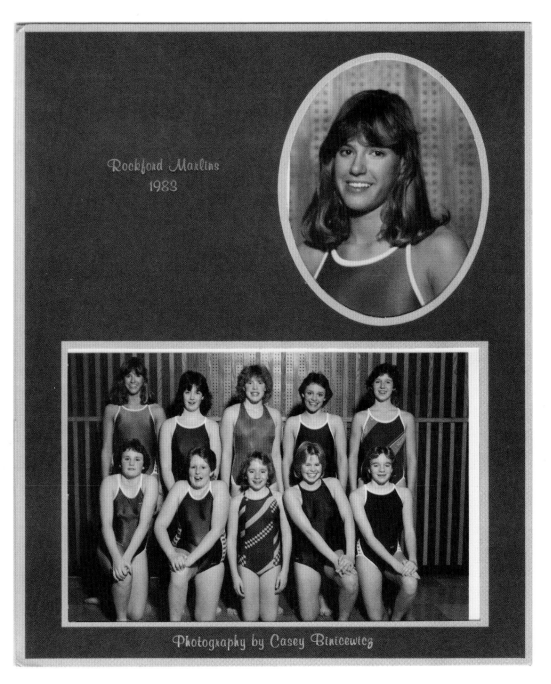

Rockford Marlins
1983

Photography by Casey Binicewicz

My high school swim team photo. PHOTO BY CASEY BINICEWICZ

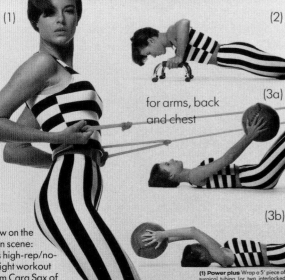

New on the
lean scene:
this high-rep/no-
weight workout
from Cara Sax of
The Trainer's Edge,
NYC. The key concept?
The "superset"—2 to 3 high-
intensity exercises you do
in tandem to tone and
elongate specific muscle
groups. Do each superset
twice, without stopping;
the whole routine, three
times a week—and learn
the secrets of sleek!

and strong

for arms, back
and chest

(1) **Power plus** Wrap a 5' piece of
surgical tubing (or two interlocked
exercise rubber bands) around a
doorknob, tie a loop at each end.
Stand with feet shoulder-width apart,
knees slightly bent and grasp loops,
palms up, arms straight out in front,
back straight and tummy pulled in.
Slowly pull tubing to waist; return to
starting position. Do 20 times.
(2) **Push-ups plus** Lie facedown,
knees bent and lower legs off floor;
set push-up bars (or use propped-up
encyclopedias) slightly more than
shoulder-width apart. Hold on to
bars with arms extended. With back
straight, lower
exhale and strai
back up. Do 20
(3) **Pullover**
knees bent on
apart, feet off fl
ber ball above
bent. (b) Keepi
slowly extend a
until the ball to
bring it forward
Crop top, $22, leggings,
by Dance Basics, NY. Aer
wear, $49.95. Tubing av
Push-up bars available
see SHOP.

This early modeling job
looks much different—and
much funnier—than my
cover article in *Shape*
magazine's September
2011 issue. Can you
believe the clothes? Or
the exercises? COURTESY OF
CONDE NAST ARCHIVES

An early modeling job.

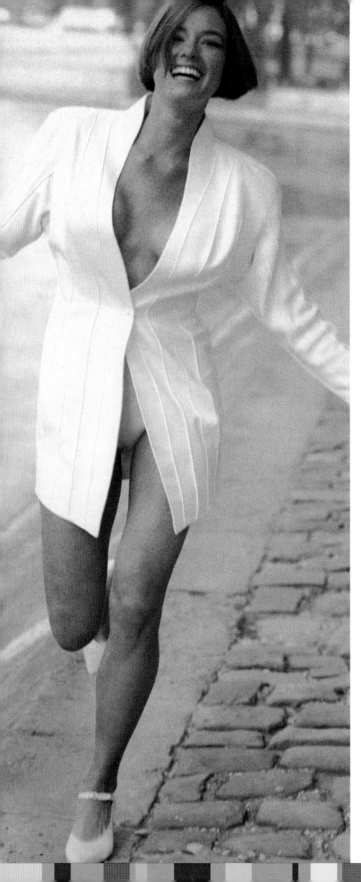

I have a full, athletic body in this Spanish *Vogue* shoot. PHOTO BY BICO STUPAKOFF

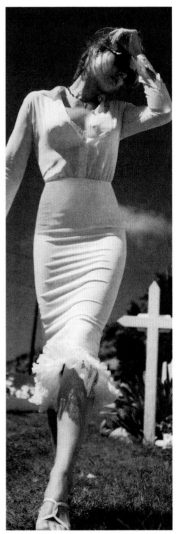

Modeling for Gilles in St. Bart's after a no-carb diet. I felt faint and had no energy. PHOTO BY GILLES BENSIMON

All-American Girl.

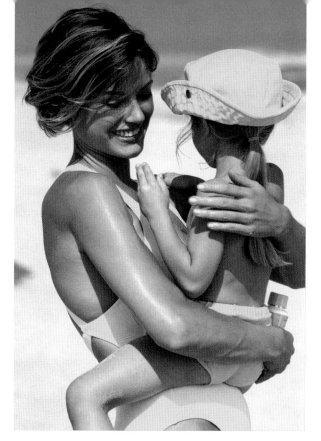

A Clarins campaign. My body was a little fuller after I had my first daughter, Sea.

PHOTO BY GILLES BENSIMON

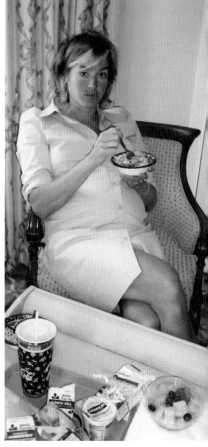

Pregnant with Sea.

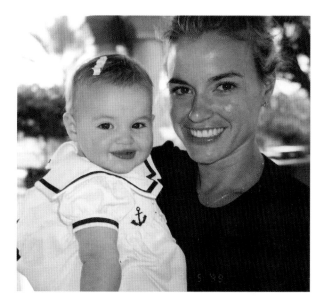

Me and beautiful baby Sea.

PHOTO BY GILLES BENSIMON

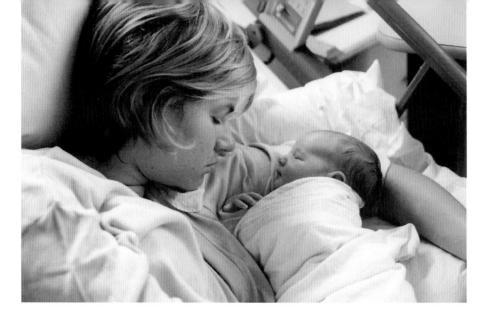

Meeting Sea just after she was born. PHOTO BY GILLES BENSIMON

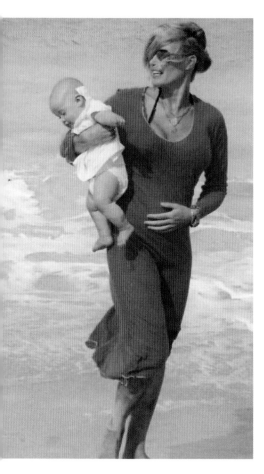

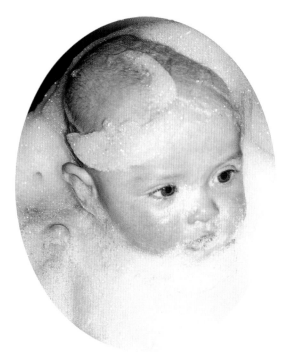

Here's Teddy in the tub—one of the inspirations for the "Babylove" smoothie recipe. PHOTO BY GILLES BENSIMON

Five months after I had Teddy, I'm carrying her—and a little bit of baby weight! PHOTO BY GILLES BENSIMON

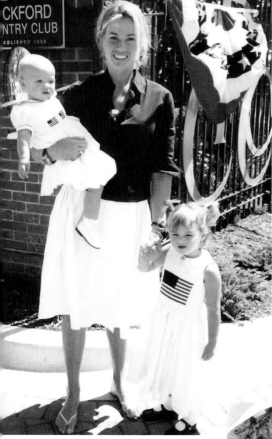

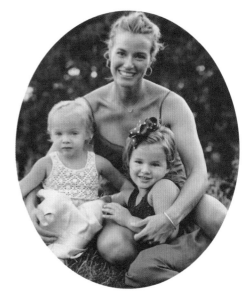

Enjoying the outdoors with Teddy and Sea. PHOTO BY MATT ALBIANI

Out and about with my girls.

Fun with Sea and Teddy.
COURTESY OF ATLANTIS

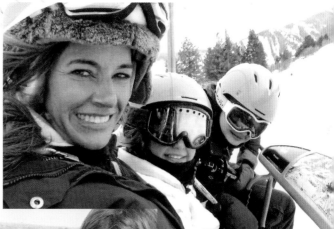

Heading up the mountain!

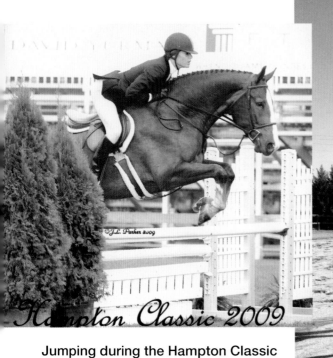

Hampton Classic 2009

Jumping during the Hampton Classic 2009. Riding horses is such amazing exercise, and I love it!

COURTESY OF JAMES L. PARKER PHOTOGRAPHY

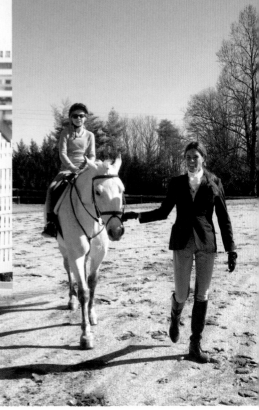

Teddy taking her turn.

Sea, Teddy, and me taking a bicycle ride with our dogs (left to right) Bear, Fluffy, and Chief. PHOTO BY MATT ALBIANI

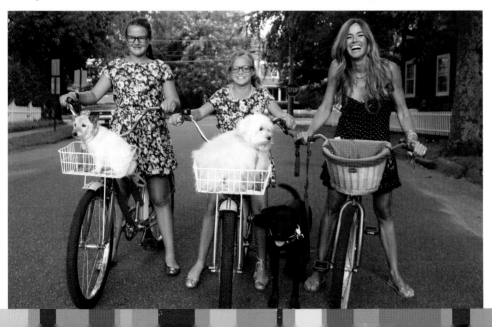

Staying hydrated is important no matter what you're doing, so I always try to drink eight glasses or about a liter of water a day. Soda isn't water. Coffee isn't water. Water is water. Drink throughout the day; don't try to get it all down at once. You wouldn't drown an orchid, so don't drown yourself.

Even when I was training to run the New York City Marathon in 2007, I stuck to my basic diet. I ate high-fiber cereal for breakfast, lots of good carbs for lunch, and a steak and salad for dinner. I didn't stuff myself (even at the carb-loading fest at Tavern on the Green the night before when everyone around me was loading up on pasta and beer), and when I completed the run—on the first day of my period, I should add—I felt fit and strong rather than depleted.

That said, however, everyone, including me, has some days when their energy is not as high as they would like or need

H*tip*T

Sometimes when you think you are hungry, you really just need a little energy boost and a sweet drink will do the trick. Next time you think you're hungry, try a lemonade and a diversion.

it to be in order to get everything done. I don't have a life that allows me to crash and burn, so here are a few of the energy boosters I reach for when I'm having one of those days:

- **JELLY BEANS: Find really good ones that are so bursting with great flavor that you really can't eat more than a few. They're tiny, they satisfy my sweet tooth, and they give me that burst of energy I need to keep on going. At that point, I'm frankly not concerned with sugar turning to fat. I just know what I need.**

- **GOJI BERRIES:** They have many different nutrients and antioxidants to help boost my immune system and keep me looking and feeling HOT.

- Dehydrated fruit of any kind

- Frozen grapes

- Tomato, pineapple, cantaloupe, or watermelon with a dash of salt

- Peanut butter on rice crackers

- Jicama (a great substitute for chips) with guacamole

- Hummus with baked tortilla chips

Kelly's Cardinal Rule

Even though I do drink Diet Coke, when it comes to food, I'd rather have you stick to your sugar instead of artificial sweeteners and get more spice (or sweet) out of life.

Remember that hot isn't just *caliente*; it's also spicy and sultry. Red hot condiments can spice up your food and jump-start your metabolism without adding many calories. Here are a few of my favorites:

h⊙t button issue

We keep reading about how bad sodium is for our health, but if you eat fresh foods that you prepare yourself, you can determine and control the amount of salt you want to use. I, Kelly Killoren Bensimon, am perfectly capable of deciding how much salt I want to put on my food. I don't need anyone else to salt my food for me. I know that the amount of salt I choose to sprinkle on my food is not going to hurt me. As a general rule of thumb, taste first, salt after.

KELLY'S RED-HOT FOOD LIST

- Baked corn tortillas with paprika

- Baked potato skins with yogurt and chili powder

- Boneless Buffalo chicken wings

- Candied jalapeños (aka "cowboy candies")

- Cinnamon and cayenne almonds

- Dehydrated corn kernels with chili powder

- Hot tamales

- Popcorn with sugar and cinnamon or cayenne pepper

- Samosas

- Spicy almonds with chili powder and sea salt

- Spicy lentils with sesame seeds

- Snyder's of Hanover Buffalo Wing Pretzel Pieces

- Taquitos with red peppers, avocado, and spicy mayo

Remember, condiments are accessories that can make your food delicious; it's up to you to make it nutritious.

RED-HOT SWEET TREATS

- **Atomic Fireballs**

- **Fiery cinnamon hard candy**

- **Fiery Jelly Bellys jelly beans**

- **Hot cinnamon Flaming Hearts candy**

- **Red Hots**

- **Big Red gum**

- **Mike and Ike (all red candies)**

KELLY'S SUPERFOODS

We hear a lot these days about the so-called "superfoods" that help to lower our risk of certain diseases. I'm not a nutritionist (and I don't even play one on television) but this is a list of my own fave foods and why I like them so much—some, like spinach and salmon, are the ones that appear on everyone's superfood list, and others are my personal favorites.

- **SPINACH: It's loaded with flavonoids (antioxidants) and help to fight off cancer.**

- **SOY MILK: It's high in protein, has more fiber than cow's milk, and contains isoflavones that help prevent cancer and osteoporosis.**

- **BEANS:** They contain soluble fiber that helps lower cholesterol and slows the release of carbs into your system, which helps keep blood sugar from spiking.

- **SALMON:** It contains omega-3 fatty acids and is rich in iron, calcium, and selenium.

- **JALAPEÑOS:** The capsaicin in jalapeños and other chili peppers have been found to relieve migraine headaches as well as to fight nasal congestion. Some mice studies have also found that capsaicin has killed or greatly reduced the size of prostate cancer cells.

- **KALE:** Cooked kale (and other vegetables of the *Brassica* family) bind bile acids, which can help to lower cholesterol and reduce the risk of heart disease.

- **GOJI BERRIES (AKA WOLF BERRIES):** They contain antioxidants that boost the immune system and help to lower cholesterol.

- **GRAPESEED OIL:** It's full of antioxidants and vitamin E, and can reduce bad cholesterol while raising good.

- **WHOLE GRAINS:** They are high in fiber, vitamins, minerals, antioxidants, and healthy fats, and protect against cardiovascular disease, diabetes, and other chronic illnesses. The USDA's 2010 Dietary Guidelines recommend that at least half of the grains we eat should be whole grains (such as barley, buckwheat, brown rice, and whole grain oats—and, yes, popcorn!)

- **QUINOA:** Is one of the few plant sources of complete protein. (See To cook quinoa, page 221).

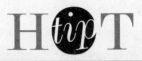

I thought I was in love with coffee, but now I think my dehydrator is my truest love. I still love to flirt with my coffee maker, but I'm wedded to my dehydrator. Not only is my entire house incredibly fragrant and aromatic, but I'm discovering taste sensations that I'd never even imagined before.

Initially I'd been buying dried fruit when I needed fun, healthy snacks to pack in my kids' camp lunch bags. Then I started eating it myself. Dried fruit is colorful and delicious. My attitude is that, if I can't make it (or a version of it) myself, there may be something in it I shouldn't be eating. So I did my research and bought a dehydrator. Mine is a NESCO American Harvest. It's not the fanciest one on the market, but it's a real workhorse. It does the job, and it hasn't failed me yet. Since then, I've been making dried blueberries, strawberries, bananas, cucumbers, zucchini, eggplant, and anything else I can think of. My favorites are snow peas, pineapple (the best of the best), apples, blueberries, mangoes, and bananas. I've also experimented with avocados, but it didn't work. Creamy, luscious avocados were just not meant to be dried. When you dehydrate fruits and vegetables, the flavor becomes incredibly concentrated; every bite packs a giant punch. Dehydrated fruits are fabulous as a snack, on top of salads, and vegetables add crunch—as in my Eggplant Lasagna (page 226). I'm not a big fan of Jerky, so I don't dehydrate meats. But if you are, by all means go for it. My dehydrator is always in use, and the whole family eats snacks that are delicious and healthy. Really, you should buy one; I promise you won't be sorry. It's really easy to do. Just slice or dice the fruit or vegetable, put in the machine, and push the button. That's all there is to it. Just remember to plan ahead, because dehydrating takes several hours or even overnight.

Now Teddy has her own "snack drawer" filled with baggies of dehydrated fruits and veggies. She can go to the drawer, pick her own snack, and I know it's going to be healthy.

Here are a few more lean tricks I've learned along the way.

- Drink a warm liquid at the beginning of a meal (try miso soup the way the Japanese diet).

- Eat a salad before a meal (lettuce has a lot of water, which will help to fill you up without filling you out. Salads also taste great, so it's a double whammy).

- Eat water-rich fruits such as watermelon, pineapple, and apples.

- Drink water throughout the day (not all at one sitting).

- Eat beans and lentils (they're high protein without all the fat of meats).

- After dinner, have a glass of water with a squeeze of lemon, lime, or a piece of cucumber in it. Lemon is an antiscorbutic, meaning that it helps to prevent disease and assists in cleansing the system of impurities. Lemon also helps with digestion and relieves feelings of heartburn and bloating. (Afterward you can rub your sink with the rind to give it a fresh, clean aroma.) The health benefits of lime include weight loss, skin care, and good digestion. Cucumber is

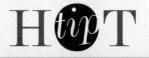

Keep a big pitcher of water with lemon or lime slices, raspberries, blueberries, or cucumber slices in the refrigerator and pretend that you're living in a very expensive spa.

**refreshing and is known as a calming vegetable that's
often used at spas. It also contains vitamin C and fiber
and helps to lower blood pressure.**

RESOURCES YOU CAN USE

Since I don't expect you to carry this book wherever you go—
as much as I would love that—here are a few phone apps and
Web pages you can access on the go to boost or reinforce your
KKBfit plan. Knowledge is key; the more you have, the better
off you'll be.

My favorite phone apps (most of them are free; a couple
cost 99 cents):

■ **Sleep Cycle alarm clock:**

An alarm clock that analyzes your sleep patterns and
wakes you in the lightest sleep phase; a natural way to wake
up where you feel rested and relaxed.

■ **Fitness Buddy: 1,000+ Exercises, Workouts, Ultimate
Exercise Journal:**

Tabs categorize exercises by muscle. Choose the muscle
mass you would like to exercise and find hundreds of ways
to do it.

Tutorials present an easy method of learning.

Built-in calendar keeps you on a practical rotation to give
each group time to rest throughout the week.

■ **Pedometer 24/7:**

Accurately measures steps, distance, calories burned,
and now has a feature to add playlists to play directly from
the app.

- **BabyCenter My Pregnancy Today:**

Enter baby's due date and the app provides day-by-day knowledge of your body's changes, fetal developments, checklist for baby preparations (decisions, appointments), nutrition guide, and connects you with other moms.

- **iMapMyRIDE:**

Uses GPS to map out your bike rides to fit your fitness goals.

WEB SITES:

- **www.amazon.com**

One-stop shopping for just about any book, periodical, or product you might want to read or buy in order to get HOT.

- **www.cracked.com**

Useful and not-so-useful information served up with a laugh on America's only humor Web site. And who can't use a laugh every day!

- **www.cspinet.com**

The Web site of the Center for Science in the Public Interest, which publishes the largest-circulation health newsletter in North America.

- **www.eatingwell.com**

The editors of *EatingWell* magazine provide information on health and nutrition as well as all kinds of healthy recipes and cooking information.

- **www.eatthis.menshealth.com**

Not just for men! Get straightforward, highly visual health and diet information from the magazine responsible for the wildly successful "Eat This, Not That" series of books.

- **www.espn.com**

Everything you need to know to stay up to date on any sport.

- **www.fnic.nal.usda.gov**

The government's Food and Nutrition Information Center, which is part of the National Agricultural Library of the Department of Agriculture will lead you to the most accurate and current nutrition information.

- **www.health.com**

The Web site of *Health* magazine provides information and recipes for weight loss and healthy living.

- **www.helpguide.org**

Helpguide is a nonprofit resource for information about mental and emotional health as well as diet and nutrition and other health issues that will help you make better choices for yourself and your family.

- **www.howstuffworks.com**

Curiosity is HOT and this Web site will give you the answers to almost anything you've ever been curious to know more about.

- **www.kidshealth.org**

The site is divided into separate sections for parents, kids, and teens to learn more about how to live better and healthier every day.

- **www.livestrong.com**

The Lance Armstrong Foundation, founded to improve the lives of people with cancer, also provides diet, nutrition, and fitness tips for anyone wanting to live a healthier lifestyle.

- **www.mayoclinic.com**

Medical and health information and news from experts at the world-renowned Mayo Clinic.

- **www.nutrition.gov**

A portal that provides links to all government Web sites having any information about diet and nutrition, including the new guidelines for MyPlate.

- **www.organic.org**

News, reviews, and sources for just about everything organic.

- **www.ota.com/organic/benefits/nutrition.html**

The Web site of the Organic Trade Association; offers information on the benefits of buying and eating organic.

- **www.self.com**

Read articles from *Self* magazine, watch workout videos, and find a calculator to help you figure out your own healthy weight.

- **www.shape.com**

Get health and fitness tips from *Shape* magazine online.

- **www.usda.gov**

The United States Department of Agriculture provides information on nutrition and health, food safety, conservation and much more.

- **www.webmd.com**

Useful, up-to-date, trustworthy information on medical and health issues.

- **www.wholefoodsmarket.com**

Product information and online shopping from the world's largest retailer of natural and organic foods.

- **www.yummly.com**

Claims to have "every recipe in the world" and lets you search by ingredient, calories, taste, price, and other considerations.

To keep track of how you're doing and how your body is changing, I suggest that you take a picture of yourself every day—not to obsess about your weight but to observe the progress you've made. Some days when you're feeling your fattest, you may be surprised to see that you really look great. And you'll also be able to notice when you need to step up your exercise or cut down on your calories. People say the mirror doesn't lie, but the mirror doesn't help you to keep a record of where you've been. Having been photographed so often has provided me with a permanent retrospective catalogue of my life—the good, the bad, and the ugly.

Pictures also point me to the looks that were good for me. They can do the same for you. Take pictures of your favorite looks and stick them up on a corkboard. That way you can see what works and what doesn't. And it's fun for both you and your friends to see how you see yourself. Also, if there's a picture in which you really look great, you can always go back to that look when you're stuck or need a quick and authentic boost.

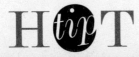

The best kind of vanity is being vain about what you put in your body.

Friday:

Hot Couture

What's hot to me is dressing to flatter your shape, whatever shape you're in. To do that you need to figure out what shape your body wants to be and then wear whatever it is that's going to flatter your figure. Just be sure it's also appropriate for the occasion. When going on a first date, a job interview, or to dinner with his parents, keep it simple. Wear basic, neutral colors and let your personality shine brighter than your fashion style. When you're with good friends who you love and trust, that's the time to take chances and expand your fashion horizons.

We all have days or occasions when we feel fat, and for a lot of us the go-to fat outfit is a great big shirt or something else big and baggy that we think we can hide behind (or under). I've done it myself, but it just doesn't work.

When my second daughter, Teddy, was just four months old, my then-husband invited me and my then-two-year-old, Sea, to come to Los Angeles, where he was photographing Madonna for the cover of *Elle* magazine. I thought it would be a nice bonding time for me and Sea after she'd been sharing me with her new sibling, and I really wanted to meet Madonna. She'd had her second baby at about the same time I did, and I somehow thought we'd bond over our recent pregnancies. So Sea and I went to Smashbox Studios in L.A. on a field trip. I even remember what I was wearing that day: a white men's shirt. My dark eyeliner and blond highlights were the only features differentiating me from a beached whale. I'd gained a healthy fifty pounds with Teddy, and breastfeeding wasn't helping me take it off. There was Madonna, tiny, flat-stomached, and wearing dark glasses. She didn't say a word . . . and then it got worse. I saw a bunch of photos my husband had shot of her in what looked like very awkward yoga poses.

So, yeah, she was (and is) HOT and cool. And even if I didn't have the post-baby body she did at sixteen weeks, I slowly lost the weight I'd gained. Six weeks later I was actually thinner than I'd been prepregnancy. Running after kids, picking up after them, and lugging car seats is the best cardio exercise and strength training on the planet. I kept the eye-liner but went with the Ava Gardner, top-lid-only look. Those raccoon eyes were necessary during my white-shirt phase, but not for being supermom.

So what's the lesson here? That Madonna had personal trainers and chefs to whip her back into shape, and I didn't—and still don't. I shouldn't have been comparing myself to her in the first place. My advice to you is: don't compare yourself to anyone else, only to your own personal best. Eat well and take care of yourself so you can take care of your kids. And, worst-case scenario, tasteful eyeliner works!

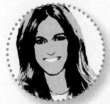

Kelly's Cardinal Rule

Let your body be what your body is and be happy with what you've got. I went to a party recently and there was Khloé Kardashian in a tight, skinny dress with this gorgeous butt you could have used to serve tea on. I have to admit, I had enormous butt envy. But no matter what I do, I'll never be that shape. It's not in my genes. Khloé Kardashian is HOT with what she's got because she owns it. I had to remind myself of that, and so should you. Stop praying for what you don't have and be grateful for what you've got.

Every body has a different shape. You need to be proud of that shape and also be aware of what your body needs. Smaller people can't eat as much as bigger people. As you get older you need fewer calories. But whatever your shape, show it off. Don't try to hide it. Hiding is not hot. It took the birth of my two girls for me to feel really good about who I was and what I looked like. Someone once told me that a woman always looks most beautiful after she has a child. I guess that's because instead of running around looking for someone to validate you, you're giving unconditional love to someone else. I thought that a "real wife" was supposed to be wearing cardigans, so I dressed down and wore bland colors. I was too insecure to wear trends. Then, when my husband and I were separated, I went back to being myself and wearing what I loved—and you should, too.

I still wear those white men's shirts, but now I wear them in my own size. So here are some of the style lessons I've learned along the way to help you determine what is the right style for *you*:

Color Yourself Beautiful

Remember *Color Me Beautiful*, the groundbreaking book that was so wildly successful in the early 80s? The reason it was (and why the Color Me Beautiful brand continues to be) so popular is that author Carole Jackson was really onto something. Dressing in the colors that complement your natural skin tones will help your inner beauty to shine through. Jackson divided people into seasons, depending on their coloring:

KKB Style Mini Manual

HOT comes in all colors, shapes, and sizes, so let's get one thing straight: When you're confident you're HOT, and what you wear can help. To maintain your red-hot confidence find the colors that work with your natural skin tone and dress to accentuate your best features.

WINTERS have skin with blue or pink undertones. They can be extremely pale, olive-skinned, or dark complected. Many Asians and African Americans are Winters. Their best colors are vivid and bold: blue whites, black, navy, blue reds, and tangerines. Metallics, such as silver and bronze, rather than pastels, work well, too.

SPRINGS have creamy or peachy white skin (the folks who tend to sunburn easily) and are typically blondes or redheads with freckles, rosy cheeks, and blue or green eyes. Springs look great in warm colors like tans, caramels, light corals, golden yellows, and light browns. Dull, dark colors tend to make them look "washed out."

SUMMERS, like winters, have skin with pink or blue undertones, but they tend to have lighter hair and lighter eyes. If you're a Summer you'll look terrific in pastels and natural shades with rose or blue tints. Try lavenders, plums, magentas, and baby blues. Black and Orange, especially close to your face, can make you look tired.

FALLS have golden or yellow undertones to their skin. They're often redheads or brunettes with golden brown eyes and olive-toned skin that doesn't burn easily. They look fabulous in camels, greens, oranges, golds, and dark brown, but shouldn't wear clothes with blue tones that work against the nature tone of their skin.

If you're unsure of your "season," hold up different colors to your face. You'll see in a minute which ones flatter and which don't. And don't be swayed by trends. Just because "brown is the new black" this year doesn't mean you have to wear it if it doesn't make you look HOT.

Hair color is also important. You can lighten it or darken it or cover the gray, but be sure the shade you choose complements your skin tone—the same way you choose your make- up. Coloring your hair isn't going to change you from a Winter to a Spring, but it can either liven up or deaden your natural beauty.

Determine Your Body Type

There are five basic body shapes—pear, apple, string bean, hourglass, and broad-shouldered—and most of us fall into one of them. If you've taken a good look at yourself in the mirror, you probably know which one you are, but you may not be so sure about how to dress in order to show it off. We can't all wear every style, but we can all find the styles that work best with what we've got.

PEAR SHAPES: SHOW OFF THAT BOOTY! To every woman who ever wanted to get rid of that fabulous behind or those curvy hips, I want to say *embrace them!* Wear shirts you can tuck in, preferably with a high-waisted skirt or pair of trousers and a fabulous belt. Try classic cropped jackets and A-line dresses, and stay away from loose-fitting tops that make you look bigger, not smaller. *For celebrity inspiration: Jennifer Lopez*

APPLE SHAPES: POLISH IT UP! Not everyone can have a waist like Scarlett O'Hara after her Mammy cinched in those stays so that she couldn't eat at the barbecue (or breathe, for that matter). I can't give you a wasp waist, but I can give you more game. Big shirts don't hide anything; they just cause people to wonder what's under there. Wear a scarf or a great piece of jewelry to draw the eye upward. Scarves are hippie chic, cool, and always HOT. Wear a square neckline to show off your gorgeous clavicles. And invest in some great shapewear. (I'm not kidding!)

For celebrity inspiration: Jennifer Hudson and Elizabeth Hurley

STRING BEANS: STRETCH IT OUT! Accentuate your thinness, not your boyish body. Wear a little push-up bra to give you more shape. You're among the lucky ones who can layer clothes without looking lumpy. Also, think V-necks, empire waists, and long flowy dresses. If you're narrow, show off how narrow you are with a monochromatic palette.

For celebrity inspiration: Rachel Zoe and the Olsen twins

HOURGLASS: WATCH OUT, CURVES AHEAD! Channel the *Mad Men* sexy teacher style. Wear sweater vests, pencil skirts, and cigarette pants. Don't hide what God gave you.

For celebrity inspiration: Sophia Loren and Scarlett Johansson

BROAD SHOULDERS: BE A LOVELY LINEBACKER! This is me. I'm athletic, lean, and have broad shoulders. I don't wear strapless, but off-the-shoulder and one-shoulder dresses look great. Go for fitted blazers, peasant tops, racerback tanks, tight jeans, and fitted shirts. I try to draw attention to my legs instead of my shoulders—for me *ankles* are the new cleavage!

Once you've figured out which celebrity most closely matches your body type, see what they're wearing on the red carpet, in movies, and at photo shoots. All these celebrities have stylists who pull the clothes, accessories, and shoes that make them look the way they do. They charge a lot of money for what they do, so why not get some free advice based on my experiences.

Look at *Us Weekly* and watch *E! Fashion Police* to see what the experts think works or doesn't work for their bodies. As you'll see, the stars are just like us, and they make mistakes off the red carpet (when they're dressing themselves), just like the rest of us.

Be Yourself, Please!

Once you've figured out the styles and color that work for you, create looks on your own by wearing things that have special meaning for you, whether it's a diamond bracelet or the macaroni necklace your kid made in school. Most important, wear them with confidence. You'll always look HOT when what you wear is an extension of who you are.

KKBSTYLE RULES

1. Save sweatpants for the gym.

2. Save PJs for the bedroom.

3. Dress as if you were the boss.

4. Dress for going out only when you're going out.

5. Remember what Carrie Bradshaw says: "Nothing is casual anymore, even when it says so on the invitation."

6. Manolo Blahniks are a girl's best friend.

HOT tip

There are always days, particularly when it's "that time of month," that most of us don't feel so hot. We tend to feel bloated and figure we might just as well let ourselves go. But if you eat well and stay hydrated, when you're premenstrual or having your period, you'll find that the hormones don't kick in as much. Instead of eating more or going on a chocolate binge, flush your body with extra water, eat light, keep exercising,

Being shapely is HOT. Think of all the curvaceous movie stars like Raquel Welch, Elizabeth Taylor, Marilyn Monroe, Jane Russell. They're sexy, not skinny. I may look thin in some pictures when I'm coming out of freezing cold water, but normally people describe me as "in shape," not "skinny"—and that suits me just fine. I work too hard to be called skinny.

and you'll feel better because your endorphins will be flowing while your body is sloughing off unwanted endometrium and mucus. Instead of getting out the fat girl shirt, put on a tank top and a great-looking jacket or even some flattening shapewear. Even for the *Shape* magazine launch party, I wore shapewear underneath my really tight dress because I wanted to be sure all my body parts stayed where they belonged, and I wanted to look as smooth as I could. Bottom line: If you look good, you'll always feel better.

Here are a few tips for looking HOT when you don't feel so hot from makeup guru Quinn Murphy, who does makeup for celebrities Mariah Carey, Anne Hathaway, America Ferrera, Nina Garcia, Angie Harmon, and Liv Tyler, among others. He has been doing mine since I joined the cast of the *Real Housewives of New York City*.

- When you are not feeling well, you'll probably have puffiness and dark circles under your eyes. Start by applying a cold compress under your eyes. You can use cucumber slices, a bag of frozen peas, or anything cold. This will reduce the swelling. I like to keep a small test-size jar of moisturizer in the refrigerator to apply to the undereye area in these urgent times.

- When you're under the weather, your skin usually lacks color and glow. Use a cream blush in a warm, natural color followed by a cream or powder bronzer. Then apply a cream or powder highlighter to the top of your cheekbones, down the bridge of the nose, and in the center of the forehead and chin to bring back the glow and luster to your complexion.

- Eye-brightening eye drops (which I call "wasabi" because they sting) work miracles—turning bloodshot eyes ultrabright and white. Apply a few drops in each eye and roll your eyes from side to side to spread it around. The ones I like best are Rohto V cooling redness reliever eye drops.

- Another magic trick is to curl your eyelashes. Curling will open your eyes and make you look more awake. Then apply a subtle cream shimmery shadow to the lids and a coat of mascara to your lashes.

- Use a lipstick or gloss with a pop of color. Stay away from nude lips and choose something with a cherry tint.

These quick tricks will help you fake your way through any not-so-hot day:

"Red hot is always sexy!" I learned that from one of my best friends, Stefani Greenfield, who is the co-founder of Scoop, one of the hottest, sexiest clothing stores in New York and who now has her own line, Curations, on HSN, and the line Theodora and Callum. When I was pregnant with Sea I wasn't feeling very sexy and my feet looked like paws. So what did I do to make myself feel better? I painted my toenails red!

Years later, filming Season 3 of the *Real Housewives of New York City*, I cut my fingernails short and painted them red to feel sexy while all the women were yelling, fighting, and being mean to one another. I even painted my nails red the minute I started writing this book. I wanted to see my short red nails tapping away on my Macbook Pro. Almost every red dress is smokin' HOT, and I've never met a guy who doesn't think a woman in a red dress isn't hot. He's a liar if he denies it. When I was sitting in the front row of a Marc Jacobs fashion show a few years ago, I wore a full, red short skirt, a tight red sweater, and red open-toed shoes. One of the editors from *The New York Times* was sitting across from me, and as we were waiting for the show to begin I kept crossing and recrossing my legs to make him laugh. It was a long wait and after a while some guy I didn't know who was at the other end of the row, leapt towards me and screamed that he was obsessed with my *feet*. How crazy is it that red open-toed shoes and red toenails could create such a reaction. Red is HOT, even stalker HOT. Yikes!

The great thing about fashion is that you can change your style to suit your mood. What are you feeling like today? Be an indie, a rocker, a prepster, or a boho. Take a page from the past: a straight skirt from the '50s, an A-line dress with pop-art color from the '60s, a '70s bohemian, Lycra leggings from the '80s, or '90s simple chic. Be a chameleon.

Every problem has a solution, so here are some other HOT tips for heating up your image:

- **Keep it monochromatic; wearing one color, top to bottom, will make you look longer and leaner.**

- **Put on slim trousers in your favorite, most flattering color and a pair of high heels.**

- **Wear colored panties and a matching bra.**

- **Put on a pair of jeans and a white tee shirt.**

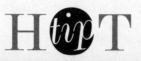

H_{tip}T

Red lips are hot, and according to makeup artist extraordinaire Quinn Murphy, anyone can wear them. "Red pouts are sophisticated, luxurious, confident, and impossibly chic," says Quinn. "If you are wondering whether you can pull off a red lip, doubt no more!"

I think of red as a dramatic neutral. There are many shades, undertones, and finishes to choose from, so that everyone can find "their" red. There are blue-reds and orange-reds as well as berries, cherries, wines, fire engines, blood, brick, and full throttle power reds—and that's just to name a few.

If you are new to wearing a crimson lip, try a lip gloss. Benefit Benetint is a universally flattering cherry balm with a hint of color. For a more showstopping approach, pick a creamy semi-matte formula in a rich shade.

The key to a bold mouth is keeping the rest of your makeup minimal. Perhaps you wear a raspberry red lip and finish the look with a touch of cream blush and black mascara.

When choosing your red, go with your instincts: feeling good with your red is the most important, and if you feel good, you will look HOT!

- Wear high heels around the house.

- Apply smokey eye shadow.

- Match your fingernails to your toenails.

- Match your nail color to your dessert—keep it sweet!

- Go to a department store and get your makeup done— for free.

- Put on an off-the-shoulder peasant top.

- Wear a form-fitting '50s-style black dress; it screams sophistication even when you want to scream.

- Put your hair in a ponytail.

- Try long tousled curls.

- Wear your jeans a size smaller instead of a size larger (just beware of the dreaded muffin top).

- Wear a triangle bathing suit.

- Put on a pair of hoop earrings.

- Match a hot color bag to your hot color shoes.

- When in doubt KISS: Keep It Simple Stupid.

Having your makeup done by a true artist can set you on the right track for being able to duplicate that professional look on your own. When makeup is done right it doesn't look "made-up." The goal is to appear as natural as possible. Here's what Quinn Murphy says about how to give yourself that perfectly made-up natural look:

As a makeup artist, the most important part of my job is to start by giving my clients the look of clear, silky, radiant skin. Without a perfect complexion, the rest of the makeup will not pop. Most people have flaws (gasp!) but with a keen eye and proper techniques, anyone can improve the appearance of their skin.

I always apply foundation before the rest of the makeup. It is the foundation of what is to follow, no pun intended. Once I perfect the skin it allows me to see the woman in a new way.

Start by applying a moisturizer that's appropriate for your skin type. Then apply a creamy concealer in the undereye area with a stiff brush. The concealer will do the heavy lifting and you won't have to apply as much foundation, resulting in a more natural look. I like to use a peachy color to correct the blue/dark undereye circles. Once foundation is applied over the concealer, it will seamlessly match the rest of the face. Apply the concealer only to the dark areas and discoloration. Usually this is in the fold under the tear duct and maybe to the outer edge of the eye for redness. Applying it in a "half-moon" covering the entire undereye area isn't necessary (and very '80s) and will add opacity to your makeup. Then apply the same concealer, or one that matches your skin tone, to any blemishes, redness, or discoloration.

The goal for natural healthy skin is to make it look effortless and not show any of the "work" that went into getting it that

H ⬤tip T

> Slim skirts and slacks are always flattering, no matter how full-figured you are. The looser the bottom the bigger you'll look. Just be sure that what you wear isn't just fitted but fits.

way. For that reason, I always match the foundation to the skin tone of the body, in particular the upper chest, or as the French say, le décolleté. Choosing a perfect foundation shade is no easy feat, but it is absolutely necessary. You may have to mix a few shades to achieve it, but the payoff is well worth the effort. The Luminous Silk foundations from Giorgio Armani have a superb color range if you are looking for a place to start. I suggest you test them in natural daylight for the most accurate light reading. Once you think you have found your shade, dot a small amount onto your décolleté. If it blends in with the rest of your skin, you have a match.

I like to use a wet Beautyblender sponge and tap the least amount of foundation possible onto the skin. Do not rub it or it will erase the concealer you just applied.

Follow with a cream blush for the most natural 'glow-from-within' look. I like rosy shades for light to medium skin tones, cola for tan, and raisin for dark. Using your ring finger, tap a small amount of blush to the apple of your cheek, and then lightly blend it back in the direction of your ear.

The last step is to set the makeup and control shine. Using an invisible powder and a small, fluffy powder brush, apply a sheer veil of powder to the forehead, down the sides of the nose and mouth, and a touch under the eyes and on the cheeks to set the makeup. If you are going for a "dewy" look, now is the time to strategically place your glow. Using your finger, apply a creamy highlighter to the top of the cheekbones, down the bridge of the nose, and a tiny dot on the forehead and chin.

Sometimes I want to add definition to the face, and pop out the facial features. This is what I call "framing the face." This also works if someone has a tan and wants their features to glow. Think of it as a modern way of contouring.

Using a powder bronzer and a domed fluffy brush, dust the bronzer on the temples and in the hollows of the cheeks, and sweep it down under the jawbone and the tip of the chin.

Finally, we come to the eyes. Smoky eyes are sultry, powerful, mysterious, and sexy. Not only were they popular in the 1920s, they are also a constant on runways and celebrities today. Many women want to try a smoky eye but are intimidated by thinking that it is too complicated. In fact, however, this style of eye makeup can be quite quick and easy to execute using an eye pencil, two eye shadows, and mascara. The principle is that it encircles the eye with a wash of color, usually with the darkest concentration of color closest to the lash line.

I will explain the technique using blacks and browns, but you can use any color(s) you like: Start with a black pencil eyeliner and trace it along the upper lash line, filling in between and on top of the lashes. This does not need to be a perfectly straight line; just apply the liner in a shape that resembles the contour of your eye. Next, take the rubber end of the pencil (or a "smudge brush" or your finger) and smudge the black line. This creates a softer defused shape and begins the "smoking."

Then, with a fluffy brush, apply a very small amount of matte black eyeshadow, then go over the smudged line you just created. Blend the shadow on top of and slightly past the smudgy liner. The trick is to build the color using small amounts of product and making them stretch. Be strategic.

Now, with your fluffy brush, apply a matte brown eyeshadow from the edge of the black powder eye shadow over the remainder of your eyelid (the part of your eye that winks). Using a flat square brush (or Q-tip), sweep the brown eyeshadow under your eye on the lower lid.

Finally, apply jet black mascara to the top and bottom lashes. That's it. You have sexy, smoky eyes!

Remember What's on Top of Your Head!

There's nothing hotter than a HOT head of hair (unless it's a hunky bald guy). Hair, teeth, skin, and nails are what define a woman's external health.

My mother always had gorgeous, long, straight hair, but when we were kids, she cut our hair really short—probably so that she wouldn't have to deal with the tangles. When I was modeling, the agency always wanted me to keep it short. It wasn't until I had my first daughter and stopped modeling that I grew it long, and now my long hair is my trademark. With long hair, you never have a bad hair day; you just have a ponytail day.

Bradley Irion, who's been styling my hair for several years, took me from bad-Jennifer-Aniston to beachy, natural, and pretty. Everyone *always* asks me about my hair. The fact is, I get to wear it, but Bradley makes it what it is. By coloring my roots their natural color (I have tons of grays), he gave me a natural look. And then the waves come. He uses a 1½-inch curling iron to curl some pieces, leaving others straight. Then he uses hairspray sparingly, which allows me to have gorgeous hair for days; it can even handle my workouts. Whatever makes your hair HOT: color, extensions, blowouts, *do it*. Drink Kelly-Green Juice and eat oysters, whole grains, eggs, chicken, beans, carrots, low-fat dairy products, and nuts—they're all great for your hair.

You only live once, but you have at least eighty years to pamper yourself and flaunt what you've got.

Here's a hot hair tip from Bradley:

"When you are eating well, it shows up in your skin, hair, and nails. When you look in the mirror and like what you see, it gives you confidence. Confidence makes you HOT!" (It's okay to feel HOT; you've earned it!)

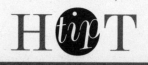

Here's another red hot tip from Stefani Greenfield (and me, too): If you want to be hot, do not dress for other women; dress for men. That means skinny trousers and high heels. It means effortless, well-fitting beauty. Men don't care about trends; they care about pretty.

"When I was working in a salon, before my client got up from the chair, I would lightly blow the hair dryer in her face. Everyone from Wall Street financiers to supermodels would instantly smile and give me a hot, smoldering look. Everyone feels HOT with a little breeze, so feel the breeze, even if the only thing that flutters is your eyelashes."

Or try one of these HOT healthy options:

- **Have a vitamin C day. Eat one fruit or vegetable that has vitamin C, such as an orange, some sweet red pepper, strawberries, or broccoli at every meal.**

- **Rinse your hair with chamomile tea.**

- **Put lavender oil in a bucket of water and mop the floors.**

- Have a vitamin D day: walk outside and get 30 minutes of sun, then drink a low-fat smoothie on your way home.

- Give the ends of your hair a cocktail of vodka, salt, and lemon juice. Then rinse, condition, put it up, and enjoy shiny sexy bed hair.

- Make sure your smile is bright and white.

- Take your bike for a spin around the neighborhood and eat an apple on the porch when you get back.

- Go out and play fetch with your dog.

- Enjoy as much watermelon as you like.

- Pack a picnic lunch of dehydrated fruit, chamomile iced tea, and mini pizzas made with corn tortillas, cherry tomatoes, and mozzarella cheese. Eat your picnic in the park.

- Chase your kids around the yard. Tuck and roll a few times, try a cartwheel if you still have it in you, then laugh all the way to the freezer for frozen lemonade pops.

- Drink a glass of water flavored with mint, cucumber, lemon, or lime.

- Come up with something fun you want to try and *do it*!

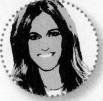

Kelly's Cardinal Rule

Your smile speaks louder than words, so be sure to take care of your teeth. Besides my hair and my legs, the one thing people always ask me about the way I look is how I keep my teeth so white. And, yes, that's also a matter of genetics. I'm blessed with the whitest teeth on the planet, and, no, I've never had them professionally bleached. But I also have tons of cavities, and I wore braces and an expander for four years followed by a retainer. Oral hygiene has always been really important to me, and it should be to you, too. Use white strips, get invisible braces if you need them, and brush your tongue as well as your teeth. *Bad breath is bad!*

Saturday: Heat Up Your *HOT* Image with Healthy Options Today

Everyone dreads Monday. Wednesday is hump day. Then there's TGI Friday. But Saturdays seem to have different functions for different people. Some people are "regroupers" who spend the day organizing their closets, doing laundry, mowing the lawn, and basically catching up on all the things that didn't get done during the week. They usually exercise in the morning and by evening they're ready to have fun and "let it all hang out." Others are "let-loosers" who couldn't care less if their closets are messy or the laundry is done. They've probably already let loose on Friday night and they're ready to do it all over again. Truthfully, I believe that in the best of all possible worlds you should be doing a bit of both.

Whether you're doing chores or just hanging out, you need to keep moving, *and* you need to take some time for yourself. Maybe in the morning you'll be doing errands or cleaning the house. Consider those tasks a form of exercise. Then have a great nutritious lunch and, in the afternoon, go for a bike ride, walk the mall, walk through a museum or a gallery, take a brisk walk in the park, or go window shopping with your friends. Do whatever it is you enjoy that also keeps you moving. Don't just wander aimlessly. If you're in the mall, go to different stores and figure out which looks will make you

HOT *tip*

Fun activities still need to be active. Keep on moving.

HOT. Ask other shoppers for advice. They have no agenda and aren't trying to sell you anything. Become the editor of your wish-list wardrobe. If you're in a museum or gallery, use the art works for inspiration. How would you redecorate your room? Is there a color scheme that speaks directly to you? Parks are great for people-watching. Who looks fit and healthy? How about a game of Frisbee? The whole world is out there for the taking so grab the gold ring. Once you're well fed you can do and be anything you want. *Nothing* is beyond your reach.

Whether you're a regrouper or a let-looser, Saturday night can be deadly if you wake up feeling bloated, sluggish, and with deep regrets on what should be your Sunday Funday. It's possible to party without looking and feeling like roadkill the next day.

We all have those nights when we want to go out, and a few drinks extend the evening into a late-night adventure. Then you wake up the next morning wondering *why* you ate those pancakes at 4:00 a.m. So eat *before* you go out. If you eat well, you'll have more energy to stay up and have fun with your friends, and you can't live on alcohol alone! So stick to your plan and *then* go out and have a few drinks. Have a glass of water for every alcoholic drink and you'll keep flushing the alcohol out of your system. You're not going to get fat from having a few drinks once a week. You will get fat if your routine is to drink, eat late, and then lie around watching television the next day, eating and making bad food choices. Going out is fun, but when you sacrifice the next day, it's never fun enough. Don't have regrets; enjoy every day. This is a life plan, and yesterday isn't coming back ever again.

If you choose to stay home, don't eat as if you were a teen-

HOT tip

Beware of buffets. Any buffet should come with a red flag warning you that it's dangerous to approach. The buffet line is an invitation to overindulge, and most of the food is dripping in sauce. Not only that, but it's probably been sitting out there for hours. Just think about that when you're tempted; it may just kill your appetite.

ager at a sleepover. If your kids are having popcorn, eat a cup, not a bowl. Hungry isn't hot and neither is a food coma.

Pamper yourself: Have a pedicure, wash your hair. It's okay to want to take care of yourself. Put lotion on your feet and your hands before you go to bed. Put cream around your eyes. Try to do this every night, not just on Saturday.

One thing I love to do with my girls is a "girls' night in."

They give me a papaya or avocado mask because papaya is rich in vitamin A, it helps to firm your skin, and is a natural antiaging remedy. Papaya alone, or mixed with milk, helps to remove blemishes and dark spots, evens skin tone, and gives you a natural glow. Avocado also has a lot of vitamin A along with vitamin C and is also great for antiaging. It firms and smoothes the skin, and because of the oils it contains, it is a great moisturizer.

We feed our hair a "cocktail" made from a "recipe" I received from Kathleen Flynn-Hui, owner of Salon AKS in Manhattan:

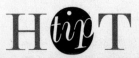

Before you get in the shower, use a trick invented in ancient Egypt. Rub honey on your arms and legs, your neck and abdomen, then wait 10 or 15 minutes and rinse it off. You'll be amazed how soft and smooth your skin feels.

Put cold and wet chamomile or lavender tea bags on your eyes when they're puffy to shrink the blood vessels.

FOR MEDIUM-LENGTH HAIR (REDUCE OR INCREASE THE
QUANTITIES FOR SHORTER OR LONGER HAIR):

> 1 tablespoon sea salt
>
> ½ cup olive oil (If your hair is colored, oil it
> judiciously, because oil can sometimes lift the
> color.)
>
> Juice of 1 lemon
>
> ½ cup vodka (optional)

Mix all of the ingredients in a large bowl. Apply to the shaft of your hair, avoiding the scalp. Let the cocktail set for 20 minutes and then rinse.

Kathleen says:

- The salt exfoliates the hair and removes build-up from product and toners.

- Olive oil is one of nature's best moisturizers. It protects hair from ongoing damage and plumps the cuticle.

- Freshly squeezed lemon juice works to lighten the hair and create natural highlights.

- The alcohol in vodka, when heated in the sun, will lighten your hair much like the lemon juice. Since we already have lemon juice, the vodka can be optional, but let's be honest, it just makes the process more fun! You can even use some of those extra lemons to make a vodka lemonade to drink while your hair sets.

KKB's Beauty Must-Haves

Airborne dietary supplements

Bliss Triple Oxygen Instant Energizing Cleansing Foam

Bobbi Brown Beach fragrance spray

Fresh Rose Face Mask

Fresh Sugar Hand Treatment

Jo Malone French Lime Blossom Cologne

Johnson's baby lotion

Johnson's baby oil gel

Kai Body Lotion

LaRoche-Posay Hydraphase skin rehydrater

Lavender flower water

Lavender oil

Neutrogena Blackhead Eliminating Daily Scrub

Rex Eme Cream

Yes to Carrots facial wipes

Zicam cold remedy

Zinc tablets, to prevent colds

Every single night I put lavender drops on my hands and rub my girls' necks. I also hold my hands in front of the dogs' noses and let them sniff. I spray my bed, my daughters' beds, and the dogs' beds with lavender. Then I make myself a soothing cup of lavender or chamomile tea. Lavender is soothing and relaxing and gets us all in the right frame of mind for a good, restful night's sleep.

People are always asking me how I manage to wake up energized each day. (And, believe me, some days I'm more energized than others, just like everyone else.) I do have a few rules that seem to work for me:

- **Don't eat too close to bedtime. (It actually takes an average of 3 to 4 hours for the food you've eaten to leave your stomach. When your body is working to digest your food, it's not relaxing, so you may find it harder to fall asleep.)**

- **Don't drink too much water late in the evening.**

- **Resolve all arguments before going to sleep.**

- **Don't watch scary movies or read scary books right before going to sleep—save them for the afternoon.**

- **Make a list of the issues that are making you stressed or nervous—and set them aside for the night.**

- **Review what made you happy that day.**

- **Think about what you're looking forward to tomorrow.**

- **Turn off your phone after 10 p.m.**

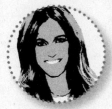

Kelly's Cardinal Rule

Wrap up every day with a great big bow and be ready for your next adventure.

KKBfit HOT Quiz

Answer the following questions to discover if you're on the right track. Did you do what you were supposed to this week so that you can enjoy your Sunday Funday?

1. **How many times a week did you have good healthy carbs for lunch?**

    Two—*not so great*

    Three—*better*

    Four—*good for you*

    Other?

2. **Are you getting enough protein? How many days did you eat chicken, fish, or meat for at least one meal?**

    I had protein for dinner every single day—*Wow! You're good.*

    I had a grilled chicken salad for dinner on three different days—*That's good, but I wish you'd get a little more adventurous in your choices.*

    I hate fish and chicken gets boring, so I probably didn't eat as much as I should—*Why not try shrimp or crab if you hate fish? Or have some good, lean red meat. It doesn't always have to be chicken or fish.*

    Other?

3. **How many days did you snack this week?**

    Two—*Awesome!*

    Three—*I hope they were good snacks!*

    Four—*Maybe you're not eating enough when you sit down to a meal.*

    Other?

4. **How many new foods did you try this week?**

None—*You need to get out of that rut!*

One—*How did that work out for you? If it wasn't great, try something else.*

Two or more—*You're really becoming an adventurous eater.*

Other?

5. **Did you try any new recipes?**

Didn't have all the ingredients I needed—*Well, next time try to plan better.*

Read through them but didn't have time—*Hope you picked one to try next week.*

Tried a couple; loved one, hated the other—*Now you've got a new one in your repertoire. Keep on trying.*

Other?

6. **How Kelly Green are you?**

I had a Kelly Green Juice—*Wasn't it yummy?*

I had a smoothie from the health food store with a splash of spinach—*Great choice!*

I had kale chips, spinach, and quinoa for dinner last night—*I bet you woke up feeling great this morning!*

Other?

7. **What are your biggest food regrets?**

Don't have any—*Really? Are you sure you're being honest?*

Skipped lunch one day and then was so starving that I really gorged on dinner—*So now you've learned something important. At least you'll be less likely to do that again.*

Ordered take-out Chinese and ate myself into a food coma—*Sorry about that, but I know what you mean. I've made that mistake myself.*

Other?

8. **How KKBfit are you?**

> Haven't had a meal since last night, but I'm going to skip breakfast and go on a run. I won't eat anything until lunch.—*Sorry, but starving your body is not KKBfit.*

> Worked out so hard, I'm going to have a smoothie—*Food should be fuel, not a reward for overwork.*

> Making pancakes with my kids, then I'm going on a bike ride—*Now that's what I call KKBfit!*

> Other?

9. **What's in your Kelly budget?**

> M&M's with a Caesar salad—*That's not enough, and I don't think M&M's are a major food group.*

> Not eating all day and scarfing a bowl of pasta—*Sorry, but that's not how to keep a Ferrari running smoothly.*

> A fruit smoothie, rice, and veggies with a salad and salmon—*Sounds like a great KKBfit plate to me!*

> Other?

10. **Which of these nutrients have you been eating more of?**

> Protein—*We all need protein to keep us feeling full and to slow down the digestion of carbs so that blood sugar stays steady.*

> Greens—*All those plant foods are filled with health-promoting antioxidants.*

> Carbs—*Good carbs give us good energy.*

> *In this case, balance is key. Just be sure you're getting enough of everything your body needs.*

11. **Which one of Kelly's recipes do you think is the most fashionable?**

> The Vogue Salad—*Haute couture*

> The Teen Vogue Salad—*Trés chic for both teens and adults*

> Jimmy Achoo's Chicken Soup—*Always in style*

> *The answer to this one is all of the above!*

12. How many times did you exercise this week?

Two days—*At least you got started.*

Four days—*Did you feel better than the days you didn't exercise? Wouldn't you like to feel better every day?*

Six days—*You're definitely on your way to being HOT!*

Other?

13. Did you try a new form of exercise?

Thought of taking a spin class but never got there—*Try signing up and paying in advance to give yourself more incentive. Make a date to go with a friend you don't want to disappoint.*

Went to Zumba but it was too strenuous—*If you're not used to exercising, start slowly. Try the 15-minute program in this book.*

Went to yoga on Monday and put air in my tires so that I could ride my bike on Wednesday—*You're my kind of girl!*

Other?

14. Are you drinking enough?

I made sure to drink 8 glasses of water every day—*Great!*

I try to remember to drink, but sometimes I just forget—*I hope you don't forget to put water in your car's radiator.*

I drink when I'm exercising but that's about it—*Not good enough! Try harder next week.*

Other?

15. Have you been taking care of your hygiene?

I haven't had time for a professional manicure, but I've been making sure to keep my nails neat and clean—*That's terrific. There's nothing that upsets me more than seeing a woman with dirty or raggedy nails.*

I've made sure that my hair is shiny and clean, even when I'm staying at home—*I love that. Remember: Your hair is your crowning glory!*

I've been making sure to clean off all my makeup before

I go to bed, even when I'm absolutely exhausted—*Bravo! I'm sure you've been feeling much better waking up in the morning with clean, clear skin.*

Other?

16. Did you do something to pamper yourself?

Really wanted to give myself a pedicure but I was too busy taking care of the kids—*We're all busy, but doing something to make yourself feel better will make you a better caregiver.*

Took your advice and rinsed my hair with chamomile tea; I loved it—*Awesome! I love it too.*

Went for a manicure and picked a really HOT color for my nails—*Good for you! Next, try matching your fingernails to your toenails.*

Other?

17. What did you do just for fun?

Fun? What's that?—*Oops, you're in danger of missing out on what this is all about.* I was really working hard, but I made sure to spend time with my friends and family—*You're on the right track. I'm not saying you can't enjoy your work, but it shouldn't become your entire life.*

I've gotten much better at time management so that I can fit in what I *want* to do as well as what I *need* to do—*Hooray! You definitely get it.*

Other?

18. What guilty pleasure are you planning for Sunday Funday?

Wacky Watermelon—*Sounds good. Just don't eat the whole thing!*

Mom's Chocolate Cake—*a great choice!*

Katharine Hepburn's Brownies—*I'm sure Kate would approve.*

Other?

Remember—this is Sunday Funday, so enjoy!

19. **What's the biggest mistake you made this week?**

Hit the snooze button and went back to sleep instead of getting up and exercising—*The best way to get yourself going in the morning is to get out and get moving.*

Sat in front of the TV and ate a whole bag of chips—*Watching TV is the surest way to indulge in mindless eating. Remember Kelly's cardinal rule: Never eat while you're doing something else!*

Went out to lunch with friends and ate the whole piece of chocolate cake even though I'd planned to have only one bite—*Share and share alike is my motto!*

Other?

20. **What was Kelly's biggest food mistake?**

Going on a juice fast—*Yup, did that.*

Going on a no-carb diet for a week—*Did that one too.*

Overeating before a horse show—*Just one of many.*

I told you I've made them all!

Still need more inspiration?

Over the years I've been lucky enough to meet some amazing people, and I've asked a few of them to tell me what *they* think is HOT. Here's what they said. I think you'll be surprised!

"Their heart, and a nice ass doesn't hurt."
—ALICE & OLIVIA DESIGNER STACY BENNET EISNER

"Colors! Are hot hot hot"
—ANGELA MISSONI

"Big calves and big hands!"
—ANDY COHEN, VICE PRESIDENT OF BRAVO AND HOST OF WATCH WHAT HAPPENS LIVE

HOT—
It is not about the look,
It is not only about the charm,
It is the perfect combination:
Sweet and tough,
Sexy and reserved,
Fragile and powerful,
And definitely smart.
—GILLES BENSIMON

"It's kindness, attention, sincerity, and the way they look at you"
—GILLES MARINI, ACTOR

"When someone knows who they are, what style reflects them, and they possess the courage to go with that I find them HOT. Oh, and they don't appear to be fighting whatever stage of life they happen to be in, be it fifteen or fifty"

—GABBY REECE, PROFESSIONAL VOLLEYBALL PLAYER

Nowadays ego gets in the way of everything and no one can seem to take responsibility for any wrongdoing. We're always pointing a finger at someone else. I think there is nothing hotter than being in a relationship and having your significant other look you in the eyes and say, "Honey, you're right and I'm wrong." To me, there's nothing sexier than a man—or woman—taking responsibility. It shows that they're confident enough to admit when they're wrong when having a dispute with their partner. That's hot.

—GIULIANA RANCIC, E! NEWS HOST AND STAR OF GIULIANA AND BILL

"Confidence makes you hot."

—ADAM LIPPES, DESIGNER

Now, as you get ready for Sunday Funday, take a few minutes to think about how you define HOT. Has your definition changed or evolved since you started reading this book? If so, I'm doing my job.

Sunday:
Funday

Wake up and do your happy dance. It's Sunday Funday. This is the day you get to bend the rules and make some bad choices! Chicken wings? Great. Mac 'n cheese? Go for it! Pizza, cheeseburgers, pancakes, Chinese, Mexican? Whatever your little heart desires.

As I've said, I don't believe in forbidden foods. If you're constantly denying yourself what you love, you won't be happy. If you're not happy, you won't want to take care of yourself. So, before you know it you'll have abandoned your healthy new lifestyle entirely.

This book is about feeling good; it's not about deprivation. It's about enjoying everything, just not every day and not all day long. I would hate it if you went to Italy and didn't think you could eat pasta. I just want you to eat it the way the Italians do—as a small first course, not as a full meal.

When my older daughter wanted to lose a little weight over spring break after spending a few months indulging in birthday bonanzas at school, I put her on what I call the ice cream diet. We were on vacation, staying at the Fontainebleau hotel in Miami, and I encouraged her to eat clean, lean foods and go with me to the hotel gym to use the Lifecycle for twenty minutes twice a day. I told her she could watch anything she wanted on the Disney channel while cycling, and she could also eat one scoop of gelato every day.

The diet could have gone sour fast, but Sea loved the TV, the gelato, and the fact that we were doing it together. I'm grateful that both the experience and my daughter stayed sweet. Since that week, she wants to "eat and cook like Mommy." She even took cooking lessons with me at Canyon Ranch.

I've made a lot of mistakes in my life, but choosing to eat well has been the best gift I could ever give to myself and my kids. I don't ask them to do anything I don't do myself. I know that kids need to gain weight in order to grow, but particularly in adolescence when their bodies are changing, it's easy for them to start gaining more than they need to just because they don't know how to moderate their eating. I know there's a fine line between encouraging your kids to be healthy and making them feel bad about themselves. My goal—and I believe my primary job as a parent—is always to make my kids feel good about themselves. If they don't feel good about themselves, they'll begin to make bad choices and blame others for their poor decisions. So don't think for even one second that I wouldn't also sit on the bike next to your daughter, if that's the encouragement she needed.

I've also done the same thing with my friend and hairstylist, Bradley Irion—although he wasn't as compliant as my daughter. For Bradley, it wasn't the ice cream, it was being able to enjoy a drink or two every day.

Bradley had gone to Spokane, Washington, for Christmas and returned carrying an unwanted gift—an extra twenty pounds. Shortly after that I was invited by *Access Hollywood* to go on a celebrity golf trip to the Bahamas. I told him I'd take him with me but he would have to eat everything I ate—and nothing I didn't—and run with me every day on the beach. We had fruit every morning and then went for our run. For lunch we had a salad with guacamole but not chips. After the first day we also added rice to our lunch. For dinner we had fish and vegetables, and we also had a couple of drinks every day.

Initially he fought me like a stubborn little kid: "You're not the 'fat boss' of me! I don't have to do what you tell me!" and on and on. I just shrugged and said, "Okay, do what you want. It's not my muffin top. Wear a tee shirt on the beach if that's what you want." But, in the end, he really did want to lose weight, so he went along with me, and everyone was amazed to see the weight coming off before their very eyes. Bottom line, I'm not the food police, but I've made myself the Sven-arbiter (as opposed to Svengali) of what's HOT and what's not.

As these two stories illustrate, and as I've already said, rules are made to be broken—in moderation. If you're eating well and making healthy choices, you can have your scoop of gelato or a couple of piña coladas and still lose weight. On Sunday Funday, make a batch of Katharine Hepburn's Brownies (page 238) or a loaf of Mom's Irish Soda Bread (page 232). Bake a chocolate cake with your kids. Invite your neighbors over for a barbecue.

H *tip* T

Grilling is a great way to cook any meat, poultry, or fish without added fat, but don't stop there. Try grilling all kinds of vegetables as well as bananas, pineapple, peaches, even watermelon. Grilled bananas with cinnamon and sugar make an awesome dessert. Wear a "kiss the chef" apron like your dad used to do when he fired up the barbecue on Sunday afternoons.

Have that scoop of gelato; just make sure it doesn't turn into a quart. Don't gorge; be gorgeous! And remember that sharing is caring. If there's something you really want, share it with someone. You don't have to eat the whole thing yourself. I know you're not starving; what I'm concerned about is obesity, not starvation. And it's just not hot to belong to the clean plate club.

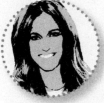

Kelly's Cardinal Rule

Sunday is for sharing. It's not a day for being alone, hungry, angry, or tired. The only drama should be happening on your television; not in your life.

There's just one rule I don't want you to break: Whatever you choose to eat, make it a dining experience. Sit down and eat a meal—and even if you order in, take the food out of the cartons and put it on pretty plates.

Sunday is also about dreaming and broadening your horizons. Read the Sunday paper—not just the news sections but all the fun sections as well—even the funnies! Check out the latest fashions. Find out what interesting activities are going on in your neighborhood.

H tip T

You'll discover that as you continue to make better food choices Monday through Saturday, your body will no longer want those "bad" things you used to crave. If you eat good food your body will respond to good food, and even your worst choices will become better choices.

Sunday is not just about making food; it's about making memories.

Get inspired by the travel section. Can you imagine going to Spain and learning to make an authentic paella? There's no dream so big that you can't make it come true.

Now, go to bed early and get a good night's sleep so that you'll be up and energized for Monday's marathon.

Just remember, Sunday *Is* Funday. Here's a couple of more things to think about trying out on a Sunday (or any day, for that matter!). You may start doing them all the time!

Why Don't You

- Make grilled cheese sandwiches or press wraps using a hot clothes iron.

- Use an electric teapot as a clothing steamer.

- Leave wrinkled clothes "steaming" in the bathroom by shutting all the doors, putting a towel under the door, and turning the water temperature up high. (You can also do this to make a mini steamroom for sweating out toxins.)

- Mix sugar with regular facewash to make a quick scrub that dissolves in water and is organic.

- Make a healthy (sugar-free) cocktail by mixing individual packets of crystal light with 1 cup soda water, 1 shot of vodka, and ice.

- Run your wrists under cold water when you start crying from chopping an onion.

- Be your own makeup artist and create tinted moisturizers by mixing a drop of foundation with a pump of face lotion (bonus points for sunscreen!)

- Use a little scented lotion as hair creme to tame flyaways and frizz.

- Instead of wiping lip balm off your fingers, rub it into your cuticles or elbows.

- Take vitamin D and fish oil to keep your skin looking bright.

Hot Recipes
for a Hotter
You

People who don't know me, or who know me only from watching the *Real Housewives of New York City*, probably think I eat out all the time. I really eat out much less than you might think. Yes, I go to many parties, events, and charitable fundraisers, but normally I don't eat at those events. I actually eat with my girls before I go out. And when I do eat out, I make sure it's someplace special. I don't just go out to "grab a bite." In fact, I never "grab" food.

Once you start eating hors d'oeuvres and drinking a few glasses of wine, your best-laid plans are bound to fly out the window and you'll just wake up feeling logy and tired the next day. Since I have a good meal before leaving home, I'm not hungry and I'm not tempted. Sure, I'll have a glass of wine. But I'll also mingle and enjoy meeting people instead of planting myself in front of the bar or the buffet table.

No one on earth would ever call me a chef. In my real life, what I am is a mom, and as a mother I'm responsible for nurturing my kids and providing them with the healthiest start that I can. I do that with good food choices and confidence-building. Balance is what I seek for both myself and my girls.

On a lighter note, it's really, really fun to cook with kids. We're in the kitchen together, measuring, laughing, and learning together. All my recipes are kid friendly. If my kids can't make them, I'm not making them. The girls get to learn math from measuring ingredients, and they also get to understand that there are some things in life you can "eyeball."

As you read through this chapter, you'll see that my tastes are very eclectic. I'm also lucky enough to be friendly with some awesome chefs who have graciously agreed to contribute recipes to this chapter, and both my taste buds and I are eternally grateful to them for both their genius and their generosity.

Breakfasts

My Favorite Cereal

I'm not a big fan of cereal, and I literally feel fat when I read what's on most cereal labels. But I can't deny my girls this classic childhood breakfast, so I came up with my own cereal concoction that contains everything I love and everything my body needs to do what it's supposed to do in the morning. Make the mixture in advance and store it in a jar or Ziploc bag for up to two weeks to cook up whenever you want. Add the dehydrated fruit just before serving.

MAKES 8 SERVINGS

7 cups quick-cooking oats

1 cup wheat germ

1 cup wheat bran

½ cup honey or agave nectar (see footnote on page 163)

½ cup water

1 tablespoon pure vanilla extract

1 teaspoon ground cinnamon (optional)

1 teaspoon freshly grated nutmeg (optional)

1 teaspoon fine sea salt

2 cups dehydrated blueberries and strawberries

Preheat oven to 275° F.

In a large bowl, combine the oats, wheat germ, and wheat bran and mix well.

In a medium bowl, combine the honey and water. Mix in the vanilla, cinnamon, nutmeg, and salt. Stir the honey-water mixture into the oat mixture until it is evenly moist. Transfer to a large, shallow baking dish or rimmed baking sheet.

Bake for 45 minutes, stirring every 15 minutes, until lightly brown. Add the dehydrated fruit and serve.

Scrambled Eggs with Spinach–Teddy's Breakfast of Champions

This is my younger daughter Teddy's favorite breakfast. She always asks for it on her birthday. Putting the frozen spinach directly into the hot eggs allows it to melt but not turn to mush. It's delicious. You really need to try it.

MAKES 2 SERVINGS

4 large eggs

2 tablespoons soy or coconut milk

One half of a 12-ounce package frozen spinach, thawed

Spray an 8-inch frying pan with organic nonstick cooking spray and heat the pan over medium heat.

While the pan is heating, beat the eggs and milk together in a bowl. Pour the eggs into the hot pan, lay the spinach on top, and scramble.

always use a nonstick pan

When you use nonstick pans you also use a lot less oil, which means a lot less fat in your food.

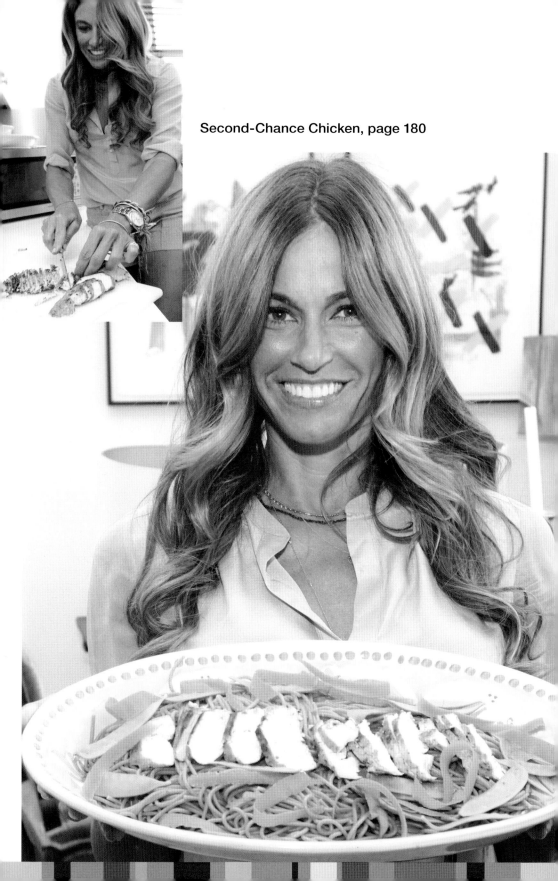

Second-Chance Chicken, page 180

You know I love both beer and chicken wings! What could be better than bringing them together?

Drunken Wings, page 186

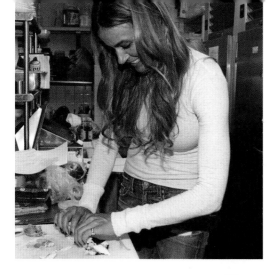

Sushi Burritos,
page 188

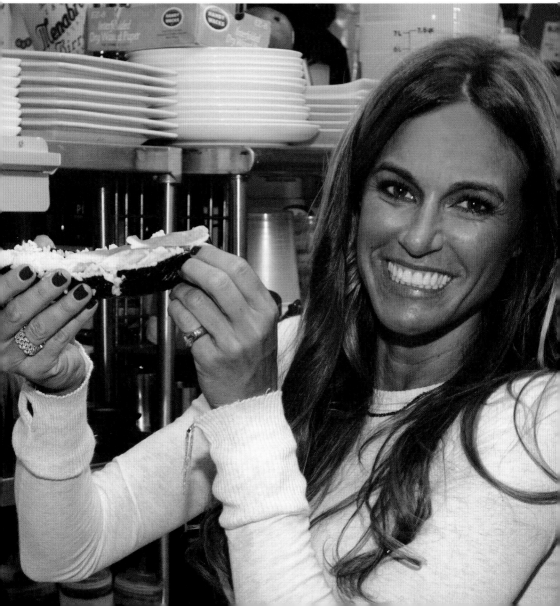

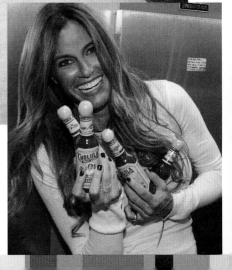

Spicy Sultry Shrimp and
Mango Stir-Fry, page 190

Hot sauce can light a fire
under your metabolism!

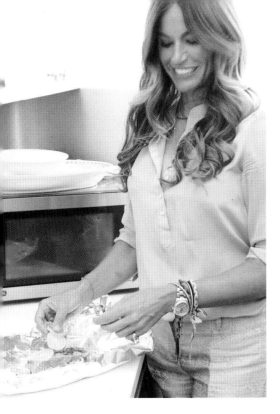

Easy Baked Salmon (without the fennel), page 200

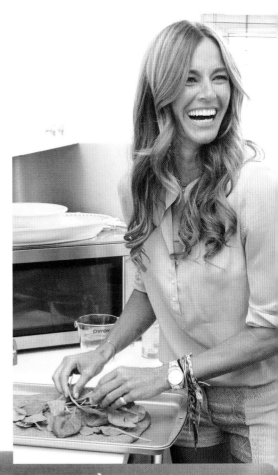

Pink Pizza, page 206

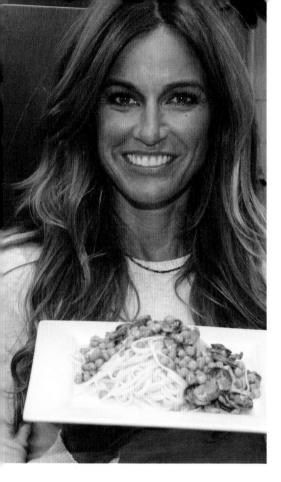

Bar No-Pitti Pasta, page 208

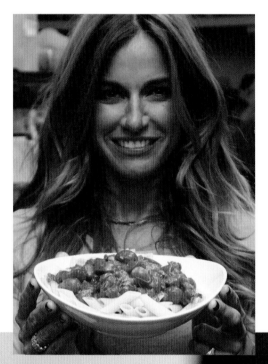

Pasta with Oddkavodka
Sauce, page 212

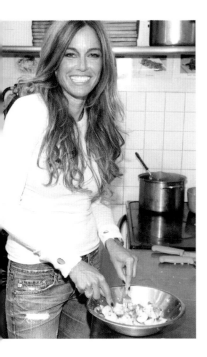

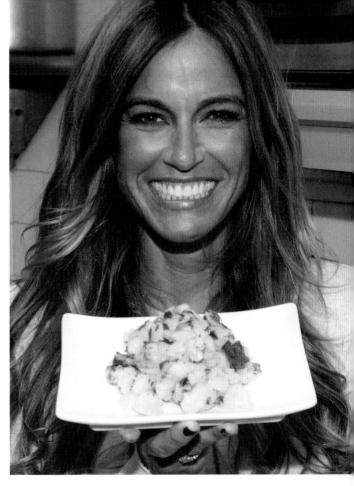

Crazy Crushed
Potatoes, page 216

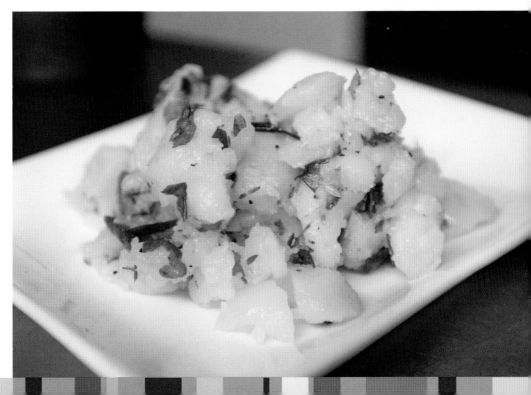

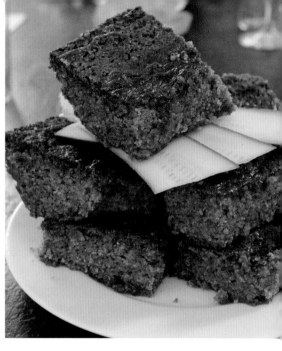
Where's the Zucchini? Bread, page 234

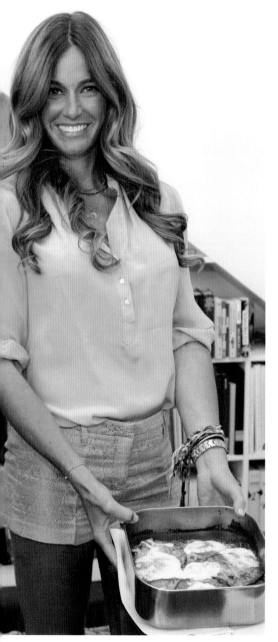

Eggplant Lasagna, page 226

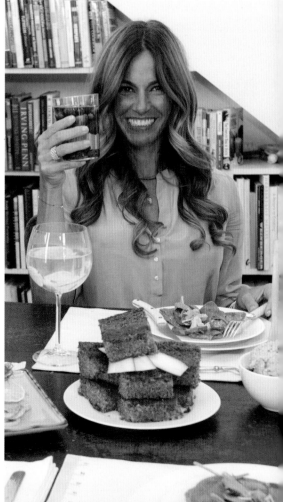

Extra-Easy Oatmeal

When I was looking for more fun recipes to try with my girls, I came up with this one—it's about the easiest recipe on earth. The kids have been eating it every morning before going off to camp ever since. It's also great if you're cooking in a college dorm, or if you're working twenty-four hours a day and don't have time to actually cook breakfast.

MAKES 1 SERVING

⅔ cup 100% stone-ground oats (not steel-cut and no quick-cooking stuff)

Water to cover

¼ cup dehydrated blueberries

¼ cup dehydrated banana, or other fruit of your choice

Ground cinnamon (optional)

Put the oats in a large bowl and add enough water to cover it completely. Cover the bowl and refrigerate overnight (if you don't, the fruit could start to ferment). The oats will soak up the water and in the morning you'll have a ready-made bowl of cereal.

The following day, add the dehydrated fruit and cinnamon to taste, if you like, and eat the cereal cold or nuke it for a minute or two if you prefer to eat it hot.

My Favorite Pancakes

I'm not the greatest pancake maker, and I probably never will be. But what I am very good at is thinking of unusual things and then doing them. We have apple trees on our front lawn, so why not make apple pancakes with our own apples? My girls picked the apples and almost fell out of one or two trees—I'm assuming intentionally since every kid is supposed to do that, right? Our three dogs were barking madly and it was a scene out of a movie: wild hair, barking dogs, children screaming with laughter, and the overprotective and worried mother shouting, "Stop. You guys, stop!" Needless to say, we picked more than enough apples, made them into apple pancakes, and I still had enough left over for a pie, which I will save for a sequel to this book called *I Can Make You Fat*. When in pancake doubt, have fun, add fruit, and see if pancakes can be a vehicle for creating great memories for your family.

MAKES 4 SERVINGS

1½ cups all-purpose flour

3½ teaspoons baking powder

1 teaspoon fine sea salt

1 tablespoon sugar

1¼ cups unsweetened coconut milk, soy milk, or any milk of your choice

1 large egg, beaten

1 teaspoon pure vanilla extract

3 tablespoons unsalted butter, melted

2 diced apples, sliced bananas, or dehydrated fruit of your choice

In a large bowl, sift together the flour, baking powder, salt, and sugar. Make a well in the center and pour in the milk, egg, vanilla, and melted butter; mix until smooth.

Heat a lightly oiled griddle or frying pan over medium-high heat. Pour or scoop the batter onto the griddle, using approximately ¼ cup for each pancake. Cook the pancakes until lightly browned. When bubbles appear on the tops, flip the pancakes and brown on the opposite side. Serve topped with the fruit.

> VARIATION: Instead of (or in addition to), the fruit, top your pancakes with agave nectar (see footnote on page 163), honey, cinnamon sugar, or jam.

Iguana I Wanna–
Cornmeal Pancakes

These were inspired by some pancakes I had in Tulum, Mexico. I know Mexico isn't known for its pancakes; however, these were the best I have ever had in my life. They were thick, like a corn cake, and I wound up ordering them for breakfast every day after my run on the beach.

Bradley, my BFF hairdresser, was with me on the trip, and one morning as we were enjoying our pancakes, I spotted an iguana who was cozying up to our table. Bradley jumped out of his seat in terror, and once I stopped laughing, I began to feed the iguana some of my pancake. He loved it. So that's how I came to have an iguana for my dining partner instead of my friend.

MAKES 4 SERVINGS

1 cup cornmeal

1 cup Bisquick

2 large eggs

1 teaspoon pure vanilla extract

1 cup soy milk

1 banana, sliced

Combine all of the ingredients except for the banana in a mixing bowl.

Spray a griddle or a large frying pan with nonstick cooking spray. When it is hot, add the batter, a ladleful at a time depending on the size of the pancakes you want. When the batter begins to firm up, add some banana slices to each pancake. When the corn cakes are browned, flip and brown the opposite sides. Enjoy—with or without an iguana.

So Smooth Smoothie

My mom loved smoothies with almonds. She was very active and always a light eater, so even though we were Midwesterners through and through, she would sneak in some "new food options," which became the root of my own "healthy options" today. Thank you, Mom, for always taking me on a run, never criticizing me for my athletic build, always wanting the best for me, and for pushing me to be better than I thought I could be. Here's your smoothie, which I now make for my girls (but without the almonds). Sorry about that, but I never really liked almonds in my smoothies—Just not, well, *smooth* enough!

MAKES 1 SERVING

3 sliced fresh strawberries

2 handfuls fresh blueberries

¼ cup freshly squeezed orange juice

1 ripe banana

1 tablespoon of BaNilla low-fat yogurt

5 ice cubes

Ground cinnamon, for garnish (optional)

Put the strawberries and blueberries in a blender. Slowly pour in the orange juice through the top as you blend. Then add the banana and yogurt, and finish with the ice cubes. Garnish with a sprinkle cinnamon, if desired.

don't drink your fruit

I believe that eating fruit is a lot better than drinking fruit juice. Fruit has a lot of fiber; drinking juice is really like drinking a big glass of sugar. So, as a general rule, my advice is to eat your fruit; don't drink it.

Smoothies, the one above included, are made with a lot of real, whole fruit, so you can drink your fruit and have it, too!

Gr-r-r-anola

If you make this in advance and store it in an airtight container, you'll always have a healthy breakfast on hand for days when you're in a hurry.

MAKES 6 SERVINGS

3 cups rolled oats

1 cup wheat germ

1 cup slivered almonds

1 cup dehydrated banana chips

1 teaspoon almond extract

1 teaspoon ground ginger

1 teaspoon ground cinnamon

¼ cup plus 2 tablespoons agave nectar (see footnote on page 163) or an equal amount of honey or maple syrup

¼ cup vegetable oil

Preheat the oven to 250°F.

Combine all of the ingredients in a bowl. Spread out the granola in a large baking dish or rimmed baking sheet and bake for 1 hour, or until golden brown. If you like smaller pieces, stir once or twice while baking. I happen to like mine chunkier, but it's up to you.

Soups and Salads

Jimmy Achoo's Chicken Soup

Rich and Skinny Cauliflower Soup with Kale Chips

Kelly Green Salad

Supermodel Salad

Kelly Beet Salad

If You Like Piña Coladas Salad

Watermelon Salad

Christmas Salad

Ivy League Chopped Salad

Warm Quinoa Salad

Kelly's Undressed Salad Dressing

Vogue Salad

Jimmy Achoo's Chicken Soup

Jimmy Choo is, of course, a famous shoe designer, but for some reason, whenever I or one of my friends used to get a cold, we'd joke about sounding like *"jimmy a choo."* This soup got its name because of the long-standing relationship between chicken soup and curing a cold. I've added cauliflower, which I love, love, love. While everyone else seems to be trying to conceal their veggies for maximum food love, I'm putting mine out there, front and center. In fact, this soup is filled with veggie exploitation.

MAKES 10 SERVINGS

3 quarts cold water

One 4-pound chicken, quartered

2 packets Goya seasoning with cilantro and achiote

6 large carrots, thinly sliced

3 large celery stalks, sliced

3 small parsnips, peeled and sliced

1 large onion, peeled and cut into 8 wedges

2 tablespoons fine sea salt

¼ teaspoon freshly ground black pepper

6 small red new potatoes, boiled in their skins

1 large head cauliflower, cut into florets

Pour the cold water into a large stockpot, add the chicken, and bring to a boil, skimming the foam as it rises to the surface. Add the Goya seasoning, 4 cups of the carrots, the celery, parsnips, onion, 2 teaspoons of the salt, and the pepper. Simmer, partially covered, until the chicken is cooked and beginning to fall off the bones, 1 to 2 hours.

Transfer the chicken to a plate, and when it is cool enough to handle, remove and discard the skin and bones. Shred the meat and set it aside.

Add the remaining 2 cups carrots and the remaining 4 teaspoons salt to the soup and simmer, covered, for 5 minutes. Add the potatoes, cauliflower, and shredded chicken, and cook until heated through.

Rich and Skinny Cauliflower Soup with Kale Chips

I adapted this recipe from one I found on the Internet. I wish I could tell you exactly where, but I can't. This makes *a lot* of soup. It's the meal that keeps on giving.

MAKES 4 TO 6 SERVINGS

1 head cauliflower

1 quart water

1 chicken bouillon cube

2 tablespoons extra-virgin olive oil

⅛ cup white wine

Fine sea salt

1 teaspoon freshly ground white pepper

2 garlic cloves, minced

1 small onion, chopped

½ medium zucchini, cut into medium dice

4 small red potatoes, peeled and cut into medium dice

1 teaspoon saffron

Cayenne pepper

Kale chips, for garnish*

Remove the leaves and thick core from the cauliflower. Coarsely chop the florets and reserve.

Heat the water in a large pot over medium heat. Stir in the bouillon cube, olive oil, wine, salt to taste, and white pepper. When the water comes to a boil, add the garlic, cauliflower, onion, zucchini, and red potatoes. Add the saffron, reduce the heat, and simmer until all the vegetables are cooked through, 30 minutes to 1 hour. Season to taste with cayenne. Serve either chunky or pureed in a blender or with an immersion blender, and garnish with the kale chips.

my top shelf cooking with alcohol choices

I often use wine, vodka, beer, tequila, and other alcoholic beverages in my cooking because they give food a lot of flavor. And since the alcohol actually cooks off, you don't have to worry about overindulging.

*You can purchase kale chips at health food stores and many well-stocked supermarkets.

Kelly Green Salad

I have this salad at least twice a week and, honestly, I wish I could have it twice a day. It's filled with iron and tons of mint, and it just happens to be my favorite color.

MAKES 4 SERVINGS

4 cups fresh baby arugula, washed and spun dry

½ cup slivered almonds

¼ cup cooked chickpeas, or rinsed and drained canned chickpeas

1 tablespoon olive oil

½ avocado, peeled, pitted, and sliced

Crispy kale chips, for garnish

½ lime

Combine the arugula, almonds, and chickpeas in a bowl and toss with the oil. Add the avocado, distribute the kale chips on top, and squeeze fresh lime juice to taste overall.

to make any salad greener

Add some fresh cilantro, mint, basil, parsley, lemon thyme, or tarragon.

Supermodel Salad

This is great for the 3-Day Supermodel Diet (page 55) but I suggest you try it any time.

MAKES 1 SERVING

FOR THE DRESSING

½ cup balsamic vinegar

2 tablespoons Dijon mustard

2 tablespoons agave nectar (see footnote on page 163)

Fine sea salt and freshly ground black pepper

FOR THE SALAD

3 grilled shrimp

½ cup diced watermelon

2 celery stalks, sliced

1 cup fresh baby spinach leaves, washed and dried

To prepare the dressing: Combine the ingredients for the dressing and set aside.

To serve: Arrange the shrimp, watermelon, and celery on the spinach leaves on a salad plate and drizzle with the dressing.

Kelly Beet Salad

I love beets and I love using them in a salad. Not only are they delicious, but beets are rich in vitamin C, a powerful antioxidant, and are high in potassium, which helps to lower your heart rate and counteract the detrimental effects of sodium. This salad goes really well with a grilled chicken breast and looks great on the plate.

MAKES 4 SERVINGS

One 14.5-ounce package cryovaced cooked beets

½ cup shelled walnuts

½ cup crumbled feta cheese

¼ cup dehydrated cranberries

2 tablespoons extra-virgin olive oil

2 tablespoons chopped flat-leaf parsley, for garnish

Drain the beets and put them in a salad bowl. Add the nuts, feta, and cranberries and toss to combine. Add the olive oil and toss to coat all the ingredients. Sprinkle with the parsley and serve.

If You Like Piña Coladas Salad

Stick a paper umbrella in this salad and you'll think you're at a Hawaiian luau! If you crave something sweet, this is a great salad to have on the 3-Day Supermodel Diet.

MAKES 4 SERVINGS

4 cups baby spinach leaves, washed and spun dry

2 large skinless, boneless chicken breasts, poached or grilled (about 6 ounces each)

1 cup fresh pineapple chunks

½ cup sliced fresh strawberries

1 tablespoon dehydrated banana chips

1 tablespoon unsweetened shredded coconut

4 lemon or lime wedges

Divide the spinach evenly among four large salad plates. Cut the chicken into cubes and distribute on top of the spinach. Add the pineapple chunks and sliced strawberries and banana chips and sprinkle with the coconut. Serve each salad with a lemon or lime wedge—no dressing necessary for this sweet treat.

VARIATIONS: I like my piña colada salad with dehydrated pineapple for more concentrated flavor, but my girls prefer the sweetness of the fresh fruit.

You can substitute 12 jumbo shrimp (3 per salad) for the chicken in this recipe, if you wish.

Watermelon Salad

This is delicious and refreshing to serve as a side dish with chicken or shrimp.

MAKES 4 SERVINGS

4 cups watermelon chunks, seeds removed

1 cup crumbled feta cheese

2 tablespoons chopped fresh mint

Fine sea salt

Freshly ground black pepper

2 tablespoons good-quality balsamic vinegar

Combine all of the ingredients in a large salad bowl and toss well. Refrigerate for up to 1 hour until ready to serve.

wacky watermelon

This is great for a Fourth of July picnic or a summer cocktail party or dessert. Just be sure the kids don't get into the "grown-up" watermelon.

Cut one or more "plugs" in a whole watermelon and fill the holes with vodka. Refrigerate up to 1 hour until ready to serve, or freeze it for spiked watermelon ices. This will serve a large crowd because it should be consumed with caution (and not by designated drivers).

Christmas Salad

Now you can fill your plate with Christmas colors any time of year. You can also top this salad with baked salmon if you like; it just won't be quite as festive.

MAKES 4 SERVINGS

4 cups fresh baby spinach, washed and spun dry

6 fresh, ripe strawberries, sliced

½ cup candied almonds

4 ounces freshly roasted white meat turkey, sliced

Vinaigrette dressing of your choice or use the Supermodel Salad dressing on page 155

Distribute the spinach equally among four large salad plates. Top with the strawberries, almonds, and turkey. Serve the dressing on the side and use it sparingly. You don't want to drown your salad in dressing or yourself in unnecessary calories.

Ivy League Chopped Salad

Season 5 of the *Real Housewives of New York City* was all about the blondes versus the brunettes, but when we were in L.A. for the Bravo Upfront awards, both groups went to The Ivy. Nobody was getting along on TV, but everybody loves great food.

I was introduced to The Ivy on my first visit to Los Angeles when I was sixteen. It's always been famous for its star-studded clientele and is one of the prime spots for paparazzi and people-watching.* You may not know this about me, but I'm a huge star-stalker. (Well, not exactly a stalker. I don't chase people with a camera.) On that first visit to The Ivy, I hit the jackpot. Not only did I get to gawk at a roomful of famous people but also I was introduced to their amazing chopped salad, and for once I was able to people-watch to my heart's content without having to worry about stuffing huge leaves of lettuce into my mouth. This is my slimmed-down version of the salad I had that day.

MAKES 4 SERVINGS

1 head romaine lettuce

2 skinless, boneless chicken breasts (about 4 ounces each), grilled or poached

½ cup drained canned corn kernels

1 ripe but firm avocado

Fresh cilantro leaves, for garnish

Vinaigrette dressing of your choice

Tear up the romaine lettuce leaves into bite-size pieces and put them in a large mixing bowl.

Cut up the chicken into bite-size pieces and add it, and the corn, to the bowl. Peel, pit, and slice the avocado and add it to the bowl. Gently toss all the ingredients and transfer to four salad plates. Garnish each plate with cilantro leaves and serve the dressing on the side.

HOT salad tips

- There are so many different types of lettuces available today. Try different ones to see which you like best.

- Whenever you have a salad with spinach, try adding a few fresh chopped mint leaves. I particularly love spinach salad with mint, baby orange slices, and almonds. Mint and spinach are an awesome combination.

- Be sure your greens are fresh—not limp.

- Wash and dry greens well before using. Wet greens don't taste crisp and they dilute the dressing!

- When you order a salad in a restaurant, ask for the dressing on the side. You're a grown-up and you should get to decide how much you want to use.

*The Ivy also serves versions of this salad made with poached lobster or salmon instead of the chicken.

Warm Quinoa Salad

I want to thank Nikki Cascone, who appeared on Season 4 of *Top Chef,* for this fabulous recipe. Nikki says: "It's Perfect for exercise/energy because it is high in complex carbs and has omega-3 fatty acids. I have won over many kids with the addition of the orange segments." You could add salmon or chicken for even more protein. I also love to heighten the flavor of this salad with some balsamic vinegar that has been reduced by half served on the side for people to add as they choose.

MAKES 4 SERVINGS

2 cups uncooked quinoa (red or regular)

Juice of 1 lemon

1 cup extra-virgin olive oil

1 large shallot, finely chopped

1 bunch cilantro, finely chopped, 1 tablespoon reserved for garnish

Fine sea salt

Freshly ground black pepper

½ pound sugar snap peas or green beans

3 oranges

¼ tablespoon honey or agave nectar*

½ cup toasted, shelled pumpkin seeds

Rinse the raw quinoa thoroughly under cold water. Fill a 5- to 6-quart pot with water and bring it to a boil. Add the quinoa, reduce the heat, cover, and cook for about 12 minutes, or until the quinoa is at your desired texture. Pour the quinoa into a fine-mesh strainer and rinse under cold water; cooking quinoa can be compared to cooking pasta. It should be somewhat "al dente," with some crunch, but if you prefer, you can cook it a bit longer. Transfer the quinoa to a bowl and stir in the lemon juice. Drizzle with just enough of the olive oil to moisten it. Mix in the chopped shallot and chopped cilantro, and season with salt and pepper to taste.

Blanch the sugar snap peas or beans in boiling water for less than 1 minute to brighten the color and soften the texture. Remove from the water and plunge into a bowl of ice-cold water to stop the cooking, then drain. Cut the peas (or beans) into julienne, add to the quinoa, and mix well to combine all the ingredients.

Peel two oranges and cut them into segments, making sure to remove all the white pith from the flesh. Add the segments to the quinoa and squeeze the juice from the remaining orange into a mixing bowl to use for the vinaigrette.

Add the honey or agave to the orange juice and season with salt and pepper to taste. Drizzle the remaining olive oil into

*Agave is a plant grown primarily in Mexico, the southern and western United States, and South America. While it is known primarily as the plant used to make tequila, its sap is also used to make the natural sweetener known as agave nectar or syrup, which tastes very similar to honey, but has a glycemic index similar to fructose, which is much lower than that of either honey or sucrose (table sugar).

the bowl with the orange juice, whisking constantly to emulsify and make a vinaigrette.

Mix some of the vinaigrette into the quinoa and reserve the remainder to garnish the finished plate. Mix in the pumpkin seeds or sprinkle them on top as a garnish.

Divide the salad equally among four plates, drizzle some vinaigrette around the edge, and sprinkle with the reserved cilantro.

make friends with fresh herbs

Cilantro, mint, basil, tarragon, thyme, parsley—fresh herbs of all kinds add maximum taste to almost any dish without using up any of your calorie budget. And you can grow your own almost anywhere. Plant a few in little pots on your windowsill, or, if you have the space, start an herb garden. It's great to be able to snip just what you need whenever you want it.

Kelly's Undressed Salad Dressing

3 tablespoons honey or agave nectar (see footnote on page 163)

3 tablespoons extra-virgin olive oil

3 teaspoons vinegar of your choice

Fine sea salt

Freshly ground black pepper

Shot of hot sauce (If you want to get HOT!)

Put the honey and olive oil in a small bowl. Add the vinegar and whisk to emulsify. Season with salt and pepper to taste. Finish off with a shot of hot sauce, *if you dare!*

Vogue Salad

At lunchtime Anna Wintour, editor-in-chief of
Vogue, can often be spotted at the famous
Italian restaurant Da Silvano in New York City.
Whenever I was there, I'd look over at her
table and see her eating the same thing: a
salad of bitter greens and a steak. I figured
that if it worked for the ultimate fashion
maven it was surely good enough for me.
And, I love meat, as most healthy Midwestern
girls do, so it's a win/win—chic and healthy.

My favorite bitter greens are arugula,
chicory, and frisée. I'm not a fan of escarole,
but feel free to experiment.

MAKES 1 SERVING

2 cups bitter greens

1 teaspoon olive oil

Fine sea salt

Freshly ground black pepper

4 ounces flank or skirt steak

1 teaspoon chopped fresh rosemary

Put the greens in a large salad bowl and toss with the olive
oil and salt and pepper to taste. Grill the steak in a nonstick
pan to the desired degree of doneness, slice it, and arrange
it on top of the greens. Sprinkle the steak with the rosemary
and enjoy.

variation: teen vogue salad

Here's a fun, chic salad that will encourage your kids to enjoy their hamburger without the bun.

In fashion terms, it's the kid's kitten version of Mom's stiletto.

> 1 hamburger patty made with 6 to 8 ounces of ground beef
>
> ¼ cup arugula leaves
>
> ¼ cup romaine lettuce leaves
>
> ¼ cup sliced, canned hearts of palm
>
> ¼ cup sliced peeled cucumber
>
> 1 tablespoon extra-virgin olive oil
>
> Fine sea salt
>
> Freshly ground black pepper

Spray a grill or grill pan with olive oil spray.* Make your burger and grill to the desired degree of doneness.

Toss the greens with the olive oil and season with salt and pepper to taste. Arrange the salad on a dinner plate and top with the hamburger.

make 'em mini

Sliders are hot these days, but there are many things besides burgers that you can make mini. Try mini hot dogs, or how about mini quiches in individual pastry crusts. Making them mini is a great way to gain portion control!

*Using olive oil in a spray bottle means that you'll use less oil and will have more control over coating the pan evenly.

Meat, Chicken, and Fish

Grilled Rib Eye with Herbes de Provence

I first met Eric Ripert, renowned chef and co-owner of New York's premiere fish restaurant, Le Bernardin, when I was twenty-four years old and having lunch with my ex-husband (then boyfriend). I was on my way to class at Columbia University and Gilles invited me to lunch at his "canteen." I remember exactly what I was wearing—a white fisherman's sweater, a white man's button-down shirt, leggings, and black ballet flats, and my backpack was my briefcase. I was offered a "Gilles Bensimon Salad" (a vegetable salad with fish), and when I met Eric, who was in his thirties at the time, he still had dark hair. I was caught off guard because I thought all chefs were older, had gray hair, and smelled like garlic.

A few years later Eric catered my wedding to Gilles, and I'll never forget how he scolded me that night because I was the only one who didn't eat his food. He's since invited me many times to go into his kitchen and cook with him, but my fear of losing a finger by being overzealous has prohibited me from accepting. I regret not taking him up on that invitation. Lesson learned—any time a chef offers to teach you how to cook, say yes.

Eric may be best known for his brilliance with fish, but he's no slouch in the meat department either. This rib eye is stunningly simple and awesomely delicious.

MAKES 4 SERVINGS

4 bone-in, rib eye steaks (about 12 ounces each)
Fine sea salt
Freshly ground black pepper
6 tablespoons herbes de Provence
Extra-virgin olive oil

Preheat a grill pan or a charcoal grill and allow the coals to burn through for 10 to 20 minutes.

While the grill is preheating, season the steaks generously with salt and pepper; sprinkle evenly with the herbes de Provence, and drizzle both sides with the olive oil.

Place the steaks on the grill and cook until the meat is nicely charred on the bottom, 4 to 6 minutes. Turn the steaks and continue cooking another 4 to 6 minutes for medium-rare, or until a thermometer registers 120°F, or to the desired doneness.

Remove from the grill and let sit at least 5 minutes before serving.

what to do with half a cow

I love meat. I grew up eating lots of it. Not every child gets to go with their dad to buy half a cow, but that's what I did. We used to drive to Eichman's in southern Illinois to get our cow. On the way home I'd be biting my nails because I knew there was a freezer that had to be defrosted and cleaned. I was the ultimate household helper: fast, clean, neat, and efficient. I knew that if I did the job right the first time, I'd have free time to be with my friends. So it turned out that buying the cow and defrosting the fridge provided one of the most beneficial lessons I learned growing up—next to "finish strong": Do it right the first time, so you can do what you love. A simple ethics lesson inspired by a cow. And it didn't put me off meat a single bit.

Pencil-Thin Skirt Steak

Everyone looks slim in a pencil skirt, so it's only fitting that skirt steak is one of the leanest cuts of beef you can buy. Eat it up and slim down.

MAKES 4 SERVINGS

5 tablespoons olive oil

2 medium onions, sliced thin

2 portobello mushrooms (or ¾ pound of any mushrooms of your choice), sliced thin

1 ½ cups quick-cooking barley

1 cup chicken broth

2 skirt steaks, about 12 ounces each

Sea salt and freshly ground black pepper

Heat 2 tablespoons of the olive oil in a medium saucepan, add the onions and sauté until caramelized but not burned. Add 2 more tablespoons of the oil and the mushrooms and continue to sauté until the mushrooms are soft.

Meanwhile, cook the barley in the chicken broth according to package directions.

When the mushrooms and onions are done, stir them into the cooked barley.

While the vegetables cook, preheat a skillet or grill pan. Rub the steaks with salt and pepper and the remaining 1 table-spoon of olive oil and cook in the preheated pan for 6 minutes. Flip them over and continue cooking to your desired doneness.

Slice the steaks and serve alongside the vegetables and barley.

Baby Lamb Chops with Blueberry-Mint Salad

My mother loved to serve lamb chops with mint jelly, but the only kind of jelly I liked was strawberry, so I could never understand the appeal of that particular classic combination. Now I make my own garnish for baby lamb chops using blueberries and fresh mint instead of jelly. The combination is insanely good, and the salad, by itself, makes a delicious snack.

MAKES 2 SERVINGS

FOR THE CHOPS

1 tablespoon extra-virgin olive oil

4 baby rib lamb chops (about 3 to 4 ounces each)

Fine sea salt

Freshly ground black pepper

FOR THE SALAD

1 pint fresh blueberries

2 tablespoons extra-virgin olive oil

1 handful fresh mint leaves, finely chopped

Fine sea salt

Freshly ground black pepper

To prepare the chops: Heat the olive oil in a nonstick skillet. Season the chops on both sides with salt and pepper to taste, add them to the pan, and sauté for 3 to 4 minutes per side; you want them pink in the middle but not rare.

To make the salad: Combine all of the ingredients in a bowl and mash them together with a fork until well mixed.

Serve the chops with the salad on the side.

Sultry Roast Chicken

After my first horse show, Beatrice, the wife
of my husband's agent, made us the most
delicious chicken I'd ever eaten. Growing
up, my twin brother and I would go to my
parents' country club for "chicken night"
while my parents went to the symphony.
I ate fried chicken every Thursday night
for ages, and now, for the first time, I was
being served chicken as a Saturday lunch.
It was also the first time I ever had ginger
in chicken, and now I can't imagine eating it
any other way. In fact, chicken without ginger
doesn't taste like chicken to me anymore.
Beatrice was a wonderful French woman
who taught me a lot about good-tasting food
and always encouraged me to balance my
work life and home life, which often seemed
overwhelming. Beatrice, I'll never forget your
chicken or your integrity.

MAKES 6 SERVINGS

One 4- to 4 ½-pound chicken

2 tablespoons olive oil

Fine sea salt

Freshly ground black pepper

1 tablespoon peeled and grated fresh ginger

½ cup chopped peeled, fresh ginger

3 carrots, sliced

1 zucchini, cut into ¼-inch-thick slices

12 small red new potatoes in their skins

Preheat the oven to 400°F.

Rinse the chicken and pat it dry. Massage the skin with the olive oil and rub it all over with the salt, pepper, and the grated ginger. Stuff the cavity with the chopped ginger.* Place the chicken in a roasting pan and roast for about 1 hour, or until the chicken is crisp and golden and the juices run clear when the thigh joint is pricked with a small knife. About 30 minutes before the chicken is done, add the carrots, zucchini, and potatoes to the pan. Serve the chicken with the roasted vegetables.

spice up your metabolism

Any time you want to boost your metabolism, adding fresh ginger, jalapeño pepper, or anything spicy to your food is a good way to go. Spicy food is known to heat up your metabolism so that you burn calories faster.

*I love this chicken stuffed with ginger, but if you're not a ginger freak you can stuff the cavity with a stick of butter. I know it's a lot, but it makes the chicken really moist and delicious.

Snow White

I know that I talk about the importance of having color on your plate, but sometimes it is nice to go against type. So I created this healthy all-white meal the entire family will enjoy.

MAKES 6 SERVINGS

1 whole chicken, about 4 pounds

¼ teaspoon olive oil

White pepper

Organic nonstick cooking spray

1 whole cauliflower, about 1 pound, broken into flowerets

3 cups chicken broth, preferably low sodium

1 cup regular grits (I use Quaker)

½ cup soy milk

Preheat the oven to 350°F.

Rinse the chicken and dry it thoroughly. Rub the skin with the olive oil and white pepper to taste. Spray a baking dish large enough to hold the chicken with the cooking spray. Place the chicken in the pan breast-side-up and roast in the preheated oven until the skin is golden and the juices run clear when pricked with a fork, approximately 1 hour. After the first half hour, add the cauliflower flowerets to the pan.

While the chicken is roasting, bring the broth to a boil in a saucepan. Stir in the grits and whisk. Reduce the heat to low and simmer until the grits are thick, about 8 to 10 minutes. Add the soy milk and stir. These grits are intended to be like rice, so they will be a bit grainier than the usual creamy consistency.

Carve the chicken and serve it on a bed of grits with the roasted cauliflower.

> **VARIATION:** If you want to put Snow White in the forest, add a handful of fresh spinach to each plate and drizzle it with a bit of olive oil.

Second-Chance Chicken

I hate the idea of leftovers. To me, eating leftovers means that you're too lazy to start over, and I've never wanted my girls to think that we weren't starting fresh. This chicken is my way of making something that could have been old into something entirely new.

MAKES 2 SERVINGS

One half 16-ounce package spinach pasta

6 sun-dried tomatoes, chopped, or 2 teaspoons capers*

¼ cup snow peas

¼ cup steamed broccoli florets

2 carrots, peeled and diced

1 cup dry white wine

1 teaspoon honey or agave nectar (see footnote on page 163)

1 cup diced leftover sautéed chicken breasts or roasted chicken

Fine sea salt

Freshly ground black pepper

1 lemon

In a large pot of boiling salted water, cook the pasta according to package directions. Drain and place in a serving bowl.

While the pasta is cooking, place the sun-dried tomatoes, if using, and the vegetables in a large saucepan, add the white wine, and cook until the vegetables are soft. Toss the vegetables with the pasta, and stir in the honey and capers, if using. Top with the chicken, season with salt and pepper, and squeeze fresh lemon juice over all.

*Both sun-dried tomatoes and capers are salty, so you don't want to use both. If using the capers instead of the sun-dried tomatoes, stir them in at the end of the recipe. Capers and sun-dried tomatoes are actually great ways to add a salty taste without using salt.

Malibu Chicken Wraps

These were inspired by the wraps Chef Sam Talbot made on the *Real Housewives of New York City*.

MAKES 4 WRAPS

2 skinless, boneless chicken breasts (about 6 ounces each), grilled

8 large romaine lettuce leaves

8 slices ripe red tomato

Sliced pineapple or papaya (optional)

4 tablespoons Thai mayonnaise* or chili sauce or a sprinkling of truffle oil

Slice the grilled chicken breasts about ¼-inch thick on the diagonal.

Cut the ribs from the lettuce leaves and place them on four individual plates, two leaves overlapping on each plate. Arrange the chicken slices on the middle of the lettuce leaves, top each with 2 tomato slices and sliced pineapple or papaya, if you wish. Spread a tablespoon of Thai mayo or chili sauce or sprinkle each wrap with truffle oil. Roll them up and eat them with your hands.

*Thai mayonnaise isn't exactly low-cal, but it's incredibly flavorful so a little goes a long way. You can buy it at Whole Foods or at other well-stocked food markets.

Bad Girl Wings

These chicken wings are Sea's favorite. I'm sure she loves them because she knows I love wings (she's a cutie like that). What she doesn't know is that they are made with kamut flakes, but you can also use cornflakes, if that's all you have. I love kamut because it makes a baked chicken wing crunchy, healthy, *and* tasty. It has a slightly sweet flavor and contains more protein than any other wheat. Let's be honest; we eat with all our senses. To me, crunch always tastes better. I can't explain why, but it does.

MAKES 2 SERVINGS

2 eggs

6 skinless chicken wings

2 cups kamut flakes, crushed

2 tablespoons vegetable oil

Preheat the oven to 400°F.

Make an egg bath with the eggs. Dip each wing in the egg bath, roll in the kamut flakes, and place on a plate.

Spray a baking sheet with nonstick cooking oil. Place the wings on the sheet and drizzle with the vegetable oil. Bake for 30 to 40 minutes, turning once, until they are a crunchy golden brown.

Hawaiian Chicken

When I was modeling in Maui and took my girls with me, we all tried chicken with pineapple for the first time. Now I make this dish both because it's delicious and because every time we eat it we're reminded of the amazing view from our Maui hotel-room window. We looked directly out at the Pacific and the waves rolled in three at a time, every single minute. It was as if we were at a great big wave park, and after a while we laughed, wondering if they ever turned them off.

MAKES 4 SERVINGS

Flesh from ½ fresh pineapple, cut into large chunks (or 1 can pineapple chunks), separate the juice

1 tablespoon sesame oil

¼ cup packed brown sugar

2 teaspoons ground cinnamon

1 cup grated unsweetened coconut flakes

Red pepper flakes

2 large skinless, boneless chicken breasts (about 6 ounces each), cut into large cubes

1 (8-ounce) bag fresh spinach

Brown rice or fresh greens, for serving

In a bowl, combine the pineapple juice, sesame oil, sugar, cinnamon, coconut flakes, and red pepper flakes and mix well.

Transfer the mixture to a large saucepan over medium heat. When hot, add the chicken and cook, tossing for about 3 minutes. Add the pineapple chunks and continue to toss and cook until the chicken is cooked through.

Add the spinach, cook for 1 minute more, just until wilted, and serve over a bed of brown rice or fresh greens.

Drunken Wings

You know I love both beer and chicken wings. This is my version of a recipe I found for wings cooked in beer. If you're feeling a bit out of sorts after a Saturday night on the town, you can make this recipe and enjoy some "hair of the dog" for your Sunday Funday.

MAKES 4 SERVINGS

- **1½ pounds chicken wings**
- **1 teaspoon fine sea salt**
- **1 teaspoon freshly ground black pepper**
- **1 bottle favorite beer (mine is Corona)**
- **1 tablespoon chopped fresh thyme, for garnish**

Preheat the oven to 375°F.

Cut the tips off the wings, sprinkle the wings with the salt and pepper, and spread them out in a roasting pan. Pour the beer over the wings and bake for 30 to 40 minutes until the wings are browned and cooked through. Garnish with the thyme and serve.

make a "clean and neat joanna"

I love coming up with cleaner, healthier but delicious versions
of my favorite foods, and this is one of them. Of course, it's
sometimes a matter of trial and error. The first time I made
Sloppy Joes as a kid, I put in coffee grounds. You know how
much I love coffee, but that didn't work out so well. Now,
instead of Sloppy Joes, I've come up with this "clean and neat"
Joanna version: Brown crumbled turkey sausage in a nonstick
pan coated with nonstick cooking spray. Mix in your favorite
barbecue sauce and 1 tablespoon brewed espresso. Serve on a
whole wheat hamburger bun.

Sea and Teddy's California Sushi Burritos

My daughters decided they wanted to make sushi, but they seem to have inherited cooking ADD from their mom. Making the rice was easy, and taking the crabmeat out of the shells was fun, but making those precise, tightly packed sushi rolls bored them. So, we decided to make sushi burritos instead.

MAKES 6 SERVINGS

One 8-ounce package imitation crabmeat or 4 frozen king crabs legs, thawed*

6 nori sushi wrappers

2 cups cooked Uncle Ben's rice

1 avocado, halved, pitted, and sliced

If using the crab legs, pick out the meat, making sure to remove any cartilage. Cut the nori wrappers in half.

Scoop 3 generous tablespoons of rice onto each half wrapper. Divide the crab and avocado equally among the rolls and roll them up burrito style.

*If you're on a budget, imitation crabmeat is great; for a splurge, go for the king crab legs

hasta la vista taco bell

I confess: the love of my childhood life was Taco Bell. I was obsessed with bean burritos and cinnamon twists. When I was doing a little online research the other day, I discovered that my favorite food choices added up to 580 calories. Of course, at the time I was swimming sometimes two hours a day, so unless I'm planning to return to competitive swimming, I guess that means my Taco Bell days are over—unless I decide to chance Sunday Funday into Fatso Food Day. Probably not! But I do love my sushi burritos just—well, almost—as much.

mild-mannered mexican-tempeh burritos

Tempeh is made from cooked and slightly fermented soybeans that have been formed into a cake or patty. As you know, I love meat, but I also love trying new things. Cubed tempeh stir-fried with vegetable broth, onions, and jalapeños, makes a great burrito filling. Really—you should try it.

Spicy Sultry Shrimp and Mango Stir-Fry

This was one of the first dishes I made when I started to cook—as a science experiment. My "method" was to think of foods I loved and which ones I thought would go well together. I love cooked fruit, and I especially love mango. Pairing it with shrimp and vegetables tasted good in my imagination and turned out to taste even better in reality.

MAKES 4 SERVINGS

5 tablespoons vegetable oil

2 teaspoons minced garlic

½ teaspoon peeled, minced fresh ginger*

12 asparagus spears, cut into 2-inch pieces

1 medium carrot, sliced

1 zucchini, sliced, slices cut into half moons

½ yellow, red, or orange bell pepper, seeded and cut into julienne

1 cup snow peas

6 scallions, cut in ½-inch pieces

4 teaspoons Roland's Thai-style Sweet Chili Sauce

1 mango, peeled, flesh cut off the pit, and diced

16 cooked jumbo shrimp

4 tablespoons water

In a wok or a large nonstick frying pan, heat the oil over medium heat.

When the oil shimmers, add the garlic and ginger and sauté until soft, being careful not to burn the garlic. When the garlic begins to give off an aroma, add the asparagus and carrot. Sauté a couple of minutes and then add the zucchini, pepper, snow peas, and scallions. Cook, stirring, for 2 to 3 minutes until the vegetables begin to soften.

Add the chili sauce and toss to coat all the vegetables.

Add the diced mango and the shrimp and toss briefly. Add the water and simmer a minute or two. Remove from the heat and serve.

*If you don't have a vegetable peeler, you can remove the skin from the ginger with the edge of a teaspoon.

Kelly's Kalamari

The first time I ever ate calamari was when I was seventeen years old and modeling in Los Angeles for the summer. My sister came to visit me and we went to Malibu for brunch. I ordered the fried calamari and was sitting there with the little suction cups hanging out of my mouth. My sister and I were both hysterically laughing. I still love fried calamari, but it doesn't love me. Whenever I eat it, it goes right to my stomach and makes a little pooch—*eww!* So I came up with this equally tasty but totally "pooch-free" version instead.

MAKES 4 SERVINGS

FOR THE VINAIGRETTE:

2 teaspoons finely minced garlic

2 tablespoons finely chopped fresh cilantro

2 tablespoons freshly squeezed lemon juice

1 tablespoon cider vinegar

½ cup extra-virgin olive oil

Cayenne pepper

2 pounds cleaned calamari

2 tablespoons vegetable oil

¼ cup dry white wine

Fine sea salt

Freshly ground black pepper

2 whole garlic cloves, peeled and crushed*

1 teaspoon dried oregano

A handful of cherry tomatoes, halved (optional)

To make the vinaigrette: Combine all the ingredients for the vinaigrette except for the cayenne and mix well. Add cayenne to taste and set aside while you prepare the calamari.

To prepare the calamari: Cut the bodies crosswise into ½-inch-wide strips and the tentacles into bite-size pieces. You should have about 3½ cups total.

Heat the oil in a large saucepan. Add the calamari, wine, salt and pepper to taste, garlic, and oregano, and sauté, tossing occasionally, for 2 minutes. Stir in the cherry tomatoes, if using, remove from the heat, and transfer to a serving bowl. Toss with the vinaigrette.

*An easy way to crush garlic is to lay it on a cutting board and smack it hard with the side of a large knife.

Shrimp Taco Tuesdays

I conceived this dish on a drive to the Hamptons, which the locals call "the beach." When there's a lot of traffic, the trip can take up to three hours, as it did this particular Tuesday. I wanted tacos, but not just any old tacos, so I spent my time dreaming up this "ultimate taco." I happen to love hard-shell tacos, but you can also make this with soft tortillas—and call it Shrimp Tortilla Tuesdays. The cinnamon may sound unusual, but it's delicious in this dish.

MAKES 8 SERVINGS

24 small shrimp, fresh or frozen*

4 cups baby spinach

2 teaspoons chopped garlic

2 tablespoons white wine

Pinch of crushed red pepper flakes

½ teaspoon ground cinnamon

8 soft corn tortillas or corn taco shells

½ cup candied walnuts

Chopped fresh cilantro, for garnish

In a large pan, sauté the shrimp and spinach with the garlic and white wine for no more than 5 minutes—just until the shrimp turn pink. Remove from the heat and season to taste with the pepper flakes and cinnamon.

If using tortillas, lay them on a flat surface, spoon a portion of the shrimp and spinach mixture down the center, and roll up. If using tacos, just stuff them with the mixture. Sprinkle with the nuts and garnish with the cilantro.

food ready to go

For a great quick meal, fill a taco or tortilla with cooked, crumbled turkey sausage or with grilled veggies, top with mozzarella cheese, and put it in the oven for a few minutes to melt the cheese.

*If using frozen shrimp, defrost them in cool (not hot) water. This takes only a few minutes.

Eric Ripert's Fluke Ceviche

Eric says, "The sexiest food is food that you can share easily with a partner, that doesn't give you bad breath (LOL!) but does give you a tingling in your taste buds. These foods can be anything from spicy or something earthy like black truffles to something sensuous like dark chocolate." I'm not about to argue!

MAKES 4 SERVINGS

12 ounces fluke fillets, skin removed

¼ cup thinly sliced red onion

3 tablespoons chopped fresh cilantro leaves

2 tablespoons minced jalapeño pepper

Fine sea salt

Freshly ground white pepper

3 limes

Warm toast, for serving

Slice the fluke on the diagonal as thinly as possible. The slices should be about 2 inches long by 1 inch wide.

Place the fluke in a large bowl, add the red onion, cilantro, and minced jalapeño and toss to combine. Generously season the fish with salt and pepper. Squeeze the limes over the fish and toss to combine. Marinate the ceviche for 2 minutes to allow the juices to be extracted from the fluke. Divide the ceviche evenly among six chilled bowls and serve immediately with warm toast.

Mexican Dancer Tortillas

There's a great Mexican restaurant around the corner from where I live called La Esquina where all the hipsters hang out. Sometimes I just want to channel my inner hipster at home, so I make these tortillas in my very own kitchen.

1 tablespoon extra-virgin olive oil

2 pounds skirt steak

Lawry's Seasoned Salt

Pinch of freshly grated nutmeg

Four 6-inch corn tortillas

Dash of Goya Cilantro Cooking Base*

Heat the olive oil in a medium frying pan. Season the steak with the Lawry's salt and nutmeg. Add to the pan, and sauté until cooked to your taste. Cut the steak into ½-inch-thick slices.

Place the tortillas on individual plates and top with a portion of the steak. Season with the Goya Cooking Base, wrap up the tortillas, and serve.

* This is highly flavorful and concentrated, so a little goes a long way.

Tuna Tacos

I first had these tacos in Tulum, Mexico, one of my favorite vacation destinations, and they contain everything I love—pure, creamy deliciousness! And even more good news is that the recipe contains only 1 tablespoon of mayonnaise.

MAKES 2 SERVINGS

One 4-ounce tuna steak

1 tablespoon teriyaki sauce

1 tablespoon reduced-sodium soy sauce

Pinch of sesame seeds

1 scallion, white part only, minced

1 teaspoon prepared white horseradish

1 tablespoon mayonnaise

1 teaspoon extra-virgin olive oil

Two 6-inch corn or flour taco shells

2 leaves romaine lettuce, torn into small pieces

½ tomato, seeded and finely chopped

Spray a nonstick skillet with cooking spray and heat until very hot. Add the tuna and sear on both sides for 3 to 4 minutes; it should still be pink inside.

Flake the tuna into a large bowl and stir in the teriyaki sauce, soy sauce, sesame seeds, and minced scallion.

In a small bowl, combine the horseradish, mayonnaise, and olive oil until amalgamated into a dressing.

Mound the tuna in the taco shells, drizzle with the horseradish dressing, and top with the lettuce and tomato.

try tilapia

Tilapia is a farm-raised, generally inexpensive fish. You can make it delish by grilling it with some shaved fresh ginger and serve it with ginger-and-mint-infused rice and grilled asparagus spears.

Easy Baked Salmon with Fennel

This is my version of cooking in an Easy-Bake Oven. It's about as easy as cooking can get!

MAKES 2 SERVINGS

1 fennel bulb, trimmed, cored, and sliced

2 tablespoons vegetable oil

Two 4-ounce skinless salmon fillets

2 tablespoons chopped fresh dill

Preheat the oven to 350°F.

Place the fennel on a sheet of aluminium foil large enough to enclose it entirely and brush with 1 tablespoon of the vegetable oil. Fold up the foil and place the fennel in the oven to bake for 10 minutes.

Meanwhile, place the salmon fillets on a sheet of aluminum foil large enough to enclose them entirely. Brush the salmon with the remaining 1 tablespoon vegetable oil and sprinkle with the dill. Fold up the foil to enclose the salmon, put it in the oven next to the fennel, and bake for about 20 minutes more, or until the fish flakes easily when prodded with a fork.

Unwrap the fennel and divide equally between 2 dinner plates. Top each portion with a salmon fillet and serve.

fish delish

For an equally easy and equally delicious fish dish, top a tilapía or other white-fleshed fish fillet with tomatoes and basil, sprinkle with a little olive oil, wrap it in aluminum foil, and bake as you would the salmon.

Pizza, Pasta, Potatoes, Grains, Vegetables, and Sides

Pizza Mexican Style

We know how much I love pizza, but when you're raised in the Midwest with deep dish pizza from Uno, you know those pizzas can spend more time on your thighs than they do on a plate. That's why I had to modify some of my childhood favorites. I don't want to lose the memories I made while waiting in line for what seemed like hours, and fighting with my siblings, but I do want to erase the lingering caloric remnants.

MAKES 4 SERVINGS

Four 6-inch soft corn tortillas

4 teaspoons olive oil

8 ounces fresh, unsalted mozzarella cheese, sliced

12 grape or cherry tomatoes, halved lengthwise

Preheat the oven to 350°F.

Spray a baking sheet with nonstick cooking spray. Place the tortillas on the baking sheet. Brush each one with a teaspoon of olive oil, top with the sliced mozzarella and tomatoes, and bake for 8 to 12 minutes until the tortillas are golden brown.

Pizzzzzzza!

I am going out on a limb here: people love pizza! My pizza will wake up your taste buds without weighing you down. I love to make it with my kids. Who knows, perhaps they'll become chefs and cook for me in my old age. One can only hope!

MAKES 6 SERVINGS

1 pound whole wheat pizza dough

1 cup Newman's Own vodka sauce*

1 whole unsalted fresh mozzarella cheese (about 8 ounces), thinly sliced

Fine sea salt

Freshly ground black pepper

Preheat the oven to 350°F.

Spread the pizza dough as thick or thin as you prefer on a nonstick baking sheet. You can make it round or oblong—the shape doesn't matter. Prebake the dough for 20 minutes.

Remove the crust from the oven and spread the sauce thinly over the surface of the dough, leaving a ½-inch border all around. Top with the mozzarella and return to the oven for 30 minutes, or until the crust is golden. Sprinkle with salt and pepper to taste and serve hot!

*If you're in a cooking mood, you can also use the homemade vodka sauce on page 212.

Pink Pizza

Here's a way to get all your healthy food groups on one pretty (pizza) plate.

SERVES 4 TO 6

1 pound whole wheat pizza dough

1 tablespoon extra-virgin olive oil

1 cup mixed salad greens

One 10-ounce box frozen spinach, cooked and drained

Two 4-ounce skinless salmon fillets (prepare using the Easy Baked Salmon recipe on page 200, without the fennel)

Preheat the oven to 375°F.

Spread the pizza dough out on a nonstick baking sheet as thick or thin as you prefer. Brush it with the olive oil and bake for about 25 minutes, or until crisp and golden.

Remove the crust from the oven, top with the salad greens, then with the spinach, and finally with the salmon.

Seth Levine's Pad Thai

I love pad thai, and my friend Seth Levine, a fabulous chef, helped me to make these noodles healthy.

MAKES 6 SERVINGS

3 tablespoons vegetable oil

3 garlic cloves, minced

One 10-ounce package frozen, thawed snow peas

¼ of a 1-pound Savoy cabbage, cored and shredded

1 zucchini, halved lengthwise and sliced

3 tablespoons low-sodium soy sauce

1 package firm tofu, cut into cubes

3 tablespoons store-bought peanut dressing

One 12-ounce package pad thai rice noodles, boiled for 3 to 4 minutes and drained

Chopped fresh cilantro and unsalted peanuts, for garnish

In a large frying pan or wok, heat the oil. When the oil shimmers, add the garlic and sauté for just a few minutes, until it is aromatic but not burned.

Add the vegetables and soy sauce and cook for 5 minutes.

Add the tofu and peanut dressing, then the noodles, and toss well. Top with the chopped cilantro and peanuts.

Bar No-Pitti Pasta

Bar Pitti is a well-known Italian restaurant in Manhattan's West Village where on any given night you're likely to see tables filled with movie stars and media moguls, and wait for hours to actually eat this pasta. This is my version of their fabulous pasta with peas and chorizo—and you won't have to wait to enjoy it when you make it at home.

MAKES 6 SERVINGS

One 16-ounce package linguini, whole wheat or plain

2 tablespoons extra-virgin olive oil

½ cup sliced, cured turkey chorizo

One 10-ounce box frozen peas

½ cup soy milk* or cow's milk

2 tablespoons freshly grated Parmesan cheese

Fine sea salt

Freshly ground white pepper or red pepper flakes

Bring a large pot of salted water to a boil and cook the linguini according to the package directions.

While the pasta is cooking, heat the olive oil in a large saucepan and cook the chorizo until crispy.

When the chorizo is cooked, add the peas and cook through. Then add the soy milk and grated cheese and stir until the sauce is just creamy but not goopy. Drain the linguini and add it to the sauce. Season with salt and pepper to taste and serve.

a new way to store cooked pasta

If you have leftover cooked pasta (without sauce) put it in a Ziploc bag with a little bit of olive or vegetable oil. The olive oil will flavor it; the vegetable oil will keep it tasting like pasta.

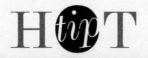

Italians eat pasta virtually every day, and it doesn't make them fat. We Americans need to learn to eat it the way the Italians do—in smaller portions, not overflowing the plate. When Americans eat pasta, we're usually having two or more portions at once without even realizing it. Please, continue to eat pasta—but only one portion at a time.

When I was married, my husband (who is French, not Italian, by the way) loved cooking pasta—especially pasta with avocado, which is amazing. He was (and still is) a great cook, but wasn't particularly interested in weight control. He'd sauté chopped garlic in olive oil, add the sliced avocado, and cook it briefly until it was slightly softened but not mushy. Then he'd season it with salt and pepper and pour the whole concoction over rigatoni.

My kids and I still love the dish, but we've learned to use portion control. We always eat this with a side salad. In fact, all pasta dishes should be served with a green vegetable or salad. That's a Kelly rule: green and white go together!

*Soy milk thickens very nicely when making sauces, but it doesn't have the vitamin D of cow's milk.

Me Love You Springtime Noodles

Refresh yourself with this Asian-flavored noodle dish. The tofu provides protein and the mint makes it dance in your mouth.

MAKES 4 SERVINGS

3 cups rice noodles

3 tablespoons vegetable oil

1 clove garlic, minced

1 small white onion, chopped

2 scallions, white part only, chopped

3 large shiitake mushrooms, chopped

1 cup cubed firm tofu

¼ cup water

¼ cup soy sauce

¼ cup chopped mint leaves

Cook the noodles in a large pot of boiling water until tender, about 4 to 5 minutes. Drain and set aside.

Heat the vegetable oil in a medium skillet. Add the garlic, onion, and scallions and sauté until soft, about 5 minutes. Add the mushrooms, tofu, ¼ cup water, and the soy sauce. Continue cooking until the mushrooms are cooked through, about 3 minutes more. Remove from the heat, toss with the noodles, stir in the mint, and serve.

VARIATION: When assembling the dish, stir in 1 cup of diced daikon radish for a bit of crunch or 1 tablespoon of sesame oil for added flavor. This dish is also great cold. After draining the noodles, rinse them in cold water, transfer to a bowl, and stir in 1 tablespoon of vegetable oil to keep them from sticking together. Cool the cooked vegetables in a separate bowl. When both noodles and vegetables have cooked, toss them together, stir in the mint, and serve.

Bowties and Green Pearls

My own inner Italian mama is extremely health conscious, so instead of meat sauce, I came up with this pasta dish made with superhealthy salmon. Not only is it supertasty, it's also superquick and easy.

MAKES 4 SERVINGS

One 16-ounce package bowtie pasta
One 5-ounce can Alaskan salmon, flaked
One 10-ounce box frozen peas, cooked
2 to 3 tablespoons extra-virgin olive oil
Fine sea salt
Freshly ground black pepper

In a large pot of salted water cook the pasta according to the package directions.

Drain the pasta, transfer to a serving bowl, and toss with the salmon and peas. Add the olive oil and toss to coat all the ingredients. Season with salt and pepper to taste.

Pasta with Oddkavodka Sauce

When you make this (especially for children) just be sure you cook off the alcohol so that you aren't serving vodka to minors or have to assign a designated driver for your guests. I always serve this pasta with a side of steamed spinach.

MAKES 4 SERVINGS

1 pound pasta of your choice

2 tablespoons olive oil

3 to 4 garlic cloves, finely chopped

One 28-ounce can crushed tomatoes, with their liquid

1 pint cherry tomatoes, halved

¾ cup skim soy milk

2 teaspoons all-purpose flour

⅛ cup vodka

Fine sea salt

Freshly ground black pepper

8 fresh basil leaves, cut into chiffonade*

In a large pot of salted boiling water, cook the pasta according to the package directions.

Meanwhile, heat the oil in a large skillet. Add the garlic and sauté a few minutes, until golden but not burned.

Add the crushed tomatoes with their liquid and then the cherry tomatoes. Cook over medium heat until the cherry tomatoes are soft and falling apart, about 5 minutes.

Stir in the soy milk and flour and cook, stirring, for a few minutes until thickened. Add the vodka and continue to cook 5 minutes more. Remove from the heat, and season with salt and pepper to taste. Serve over the pasta, garnished with the basil. If you like a smooth sauce, you can purée the finished sauce in a blender before serving.

*An easy way to cut leaves into chiffonade is to stack them on top of one another, roll them up, and slice through the roll crosswise with a sharp knife to produce thin ribbons.

Michael Ferraro's Chilled Angel Hair Pasta with Garlic, Tomato, Basil, and Parmesan

Michael Ferraro is the executive chef at Delicatessen, the restaurant where I filmed many an episode of the *Real Housewives of New York City* in Seasons 3 and 4.

MAKES 4 SERVINGS

One 16-ounce package angel hair pasta*

6 tablespoons good-quality, extra-virgin olive oil

4 ripe beefsteak tomatoes, seeded and diced, juices reserved

Coarse sea salt

Freshly ground black pepper

1 bunch fresh basil, cut into chiffonade (see footnote on page 213)

½ bunch flat-leaf parsley leaves, minced

5 garlic cloves, minced

2 teaspoons red wine vinegar

½ cup freshly grated Parmesan cheese

Cook the pasta in salted water according to the package directions until al dente. Drain the pasta, toss with 1 tablespoon of the olive oil, and spread out on a baking sheet or platter to cool. (Spreading it out will prevent it from sticking together, and it will cool faster.)

Toss the tomatoes with sea salt and freshly ground pepper to taste.

When the pasta is cool, transfer it to a large bowl and toss it with the tomatoes and their liquid. Toss in the basil, parsley, garlic, the remaining 5 tablespoons of olive oil, the red wine vinegar, and ¼ cup of the Parmesan cheese. Season again with salt and pepper.

Divide the pasta evenly among four bowls and garnish each portion with some of the remaining ¼ cup Parmesan cheese.

*You can substitute whole wheat, gluten-free, or even spaghetti squash for regular pasta if you wish.

Crazy Crushed Potatoes

These are great just the way they are—the soy milk is slightly sweet and the olive oil is a lot more heart-healthy than butter—but for something really special, add a splash of truffle oil to the mix.

MAKES 6 SERVINGS

4 medium russet potatoes, peeled and cut into large pieces

¼ cup extra-virgin olive oil

Fine sea salt

Freshly ground black pepper

1 tablespoon chopped fresh thyme (optional)

Put the potatoes in a large pot, cover with water, and bring to a boil. Cook until easily pierced with a fork.

Drain the potatoes and return to the pot. Add the olive oil, salt and pepper to taste, and mash until your arm hurts. Garnish with the chopped fresh thyme, if using.

VARIATION: Use the same recipe to make *Sweet Monster Mashed Potatoes*. Not only are the sweet potatoes yummy but they're full of vitamin A and beta-carotene, a powerful antioxidant.

kill me with kindness

I love these potatoes, but if you really want to kill me with kindness, just serve me a baked potato topped with caviar. I will literally do anything you want—within reason. I don't generally cook with a lot of fancy ingredients, but caviar is my weakness.

Yummy Yams

Yams with marshmallows are everyone's favorite for Thanksgiving and Christmas, but these are so easy that you can make them for Sunday Funday (or any day) all year round.

MAKES 4 SERVINGS

4 medium yams or sweet potatoes

½ teaspoon ground cinnamon

½ teaspoon granulated sugar

¼ cup maple syrup

1 cup mini marshmallows

Peel the yams with a vegetable peeler. Slice them in half lengthwise, then slice the halves into ¾-inch-thick strips.

Spray a nonstick baking pan with organic cooking spray, spread the sliced yams in the pan. Sprinkle with the cinnamon and sugar, drizzle with the maple syrup, spread the marshmallows on top, and bake in a 350° F oven until the potatoes are soft when pierced with a fork and the marshmallows are browned on top, about 30 minutes.

Pineapple Fried Rice

This is my own play on my favorite Thai pineapple fried rice recipe. It's what I eat every day when I was filming the *Real Housewives of New York City*. I need energy, and I crave flavor. This recipe provides both.

Try using quinoa in this recipe instead of the rice—I call that having your cake and eating it too!

MAKES 3 TO 4 SERVINGS

FOR THE RICE

2 to 3 tablespoons canola oil

3 to 4 cups jasmine rice cooked according to the package directions instead of water in pineapple juice

3 spring onions, thinly sliced

½ cup frozen broccoli florets

¼ cup vegetable stock

1 small can pineapple chunks, drained

⅓ cup chopped fresh cilantro

1 lime

FOR THE STIR-FRY SAUCE

3 tablespoons regular or low-sodium soy sauce

2 teaspoons classic curry powder

½ teaspoon dark brown sugar (optional)

2 tablespoons chopped dried lemongrass

¼ cup unsweetened coconut milk

Crushed red pepper flakes (optional)

In a bowl, mix 1 tablespoon of the oil with the rice, using your fingers to separate any chunks into individual grains. Set aside while you make the sauce.

In a small bowl, stir the soy sauce and curry powder together. Stir in the sugar, if using, until it dissolves. Stir in the lemongrass and coconut milk and add the pepper flakes, if using, and set aside.

Add 1 to 2 tablespoons of the remaining oil to a wok or a large frying pan and set over medium-high heat. Add the spring onions for about 1 minute. Add the broccoli and stir-fry for 1 to 2 minutes.

If the wok becomes dry, add 1 tablespoon of vegetable stock or as needed to keep the ingredients sizzling. Add the rice and pineapple chunks and toss to incorporate with the other ingredients. Toss in the cilantro. Add the soy sauce mixture and toss.

Remove from the heat and add a squeeze or two of lime juice. Scoop the rice onto a serving platter or into a carved-out pineapple.

spice it up

Using herbs and spices is a great way to add flavor to your food without adding calories.

Black Beans and Rice

Black beans and rice was not always my go-to meal, but when I was studying at Columbia University and traveling a lot, I lived on Fourteenth Street and wasn't keen on eating out by myself or cooking for one at home. At the time, there was a coffee shop near my apartment that made amazing beans and rice. I had already survived well on café con leche and peas in Paris, so why not channel South American culture and eat beans and rice in New York? After my morning run I'd stop in for a *café con leche,* and on my way home from class in the evening, I'd pick up an order of black beans and rice. We all know that my food pyramid is a diamond, but back then, when I was single and my phantom boyfriend was Geoffrey Chaucer, it didn't seem to matter. Now that I've started going steady with my dehydrator, I love to garnish my black beans and rice with zucchini chips. Make a big batch of this recipe and keep it in the refrigerator to heat up whenever you like. That way you'll be eating good food instead of snacking on something that isn't nutritious.

1 cup uncooked brown rice or quinoa (see below)

One 15-ounce can Goya black beans

Goya seasoning with cilantro and achiote or Tabasco

1 teaspoon chopped fresh cilantro

1 teaspoon chopped garlic

Dehydrated zucchini chips, for garnish (optional)

Cook the rice according to the package directions. (To cook quinoa, see below.)

While the rice is boiling, put the beans in a pot, mix in the seasoning, cilantro, and garlic and heat through.

Top the cooked rice with the seasoned beans and garnish with the zucchini chips.

about quinoa

Quinoa is actually a seed, not a grain, and it is one of the few plant foods that is a complete protein, meaning that it contains all of the essential amino acids that your body cannot manufacture on its own. It makes a great substitute for rice in many recipes and can be eaten on its own as a side dish or a nutritious, pick-me-up snack.

To cook quinoa

Place 2 cups of water and 1 cup of uncooked quinoa in a saucepan and bring to a boil. Reduce the heat, cover the pot, and simmer until the water is absorbed.

Barley Without the Bullfight

Turkey chorizo is tangy and lean. I love the Spanish flavor it brings to otherwise bland barley—opposites do attract!

MAKES 4 SERVINGS

6 ½ cups water

2 cups barley

2 turkey chorizo links, each about 6 inches long

2 tablespoons vegetable oil

1 leek, white and a bit of the green part, chopped

1 large Portobello mushroom, sliced

½ cup chopped fresh dill, plus additional for garnish

¼ cup freshly grated Parmesan cheese

In a large pot, bring 6 cups of the water and the barley to a boil. Reduce the heat to medium, cover, and cook for 1 hour.

In a medium skillet over high heat, combine the remaining ½ cup of water and the chorizo and sauté until the water evaporates. Add the vegetable oil to the pan and continue cooking, turning the chorizo until it is browned on all sides and cooked through, about 5 minutes. Remove the chorizo from the pan, reduce the heat to medium, and add the leek and mushroom. Sauté until the vegetables are soft and slightly brown. Remove from the heat and stir in the dill.

Transfer the barley and vegetables to a large serving bowl and mix well. Slice the chorizo ¼-inch thick and spread it on top of the vegetables. Sprinkle with the Parmesan and add additional chopped dill for garnish.

Quick-and-Easy Chunky Hummus

People tend to think of hummus as fattening, but chickpeas are low in saturated fat and high in fiber. So long as the hummus isn't drenched in oil, it makes a great snack or appetizer. Serve it with jicama chips, kale chips, baked pita chips, or try it with my baked chips. (See footnote on page 229.) It's also great as a dip with fresh vegetables such as sliced Jicama, broccoli florets, or cherry tomatoes.

MAKES ABOUT 2 CUPS

One 15.5-ounce can chickpeas, rinsed and drained

⅓ cup extra-virgin olive oil

2 tablespoons freshly squeezed lemon juice

2 tablespoons tahini

White and/or cayenne pepper

In a bowl, mash the chickpeas, olive oil, lemon juice, and tahini together with the back of a fork. The hummus should be chunky, but if you like yours smooth you can combine the ingredients in a blender or food processor instead. Season to taste with white and/or cayenne pepper.

tasty toppings

Both hummus and guacamole make great toppings for steak or fish. They're my version of béarnaise sauce. A spoonful goes a long way.

Have an Impromptu Pepper Party

Here's an easy way to make a quick, fun, and satisfying meal for family and friends and clean out the refrigerator all at once. Just mix and match the ingredients listed here, and add more fun flavors of your own.

MAKES 4 SERVINGS

1 each: green, red, orange, and yellow bell peppers

Diced leftover chicken

Chopped mushrooms

Cooked couscous

Cooked rice

Newman's Own vodka sauce

Grated Parmesan cheese

Crumbled feta cheese

Olive oil

Cut the tops off the peppers and scoop out the seeds and pith. Mix and match whatever ingredients suit your fancy.

Some suggestions: chicken, mushrooms, and couscous; rice, vodka sauce, and Parmesan; chicken, feta, and a bit of oil; chicken, rice, and vodka sauce.

Let your taste buds run wild and make each one different if you like.

Stuff the peppers with the mixture(s) of your choice. Spray a pan with organic nonstick cooking spray, stand the stuffed peppers in the pan, and bake in a 350° F oven for 30 to 40 minutes, until the peppers are soft and the filling is browned on top.

Eggplant Lasagna

I came up with this recipe one day when I was trying to think of a fun, healthy dish for my girls. I added the dehydrated eggplant because, as you know, I'm in *love* with my dehydrator, and I also love the added crunch.

MAKES 6 SERVINGS

3 garlic cloves, minced

1 pint cherry tomatoes

One 15.5-ounce jar Newman's Own vodka sauce, or use the homemade sauce on page 212

1 medium eggplant, sliced about ¼-inch thich

4 ounces shredded part-skim mozzarella cheese

2 tablespoons freshly grated Parmesan cheese

½ cup chopped dehydrated eggplant, for garnish

Preheat the oven to 350°F.

Spray a nonstick frying pan with nonstick cooking spray. Add the chopped garlic to the pan and cook, stirring frequently, for 3 to 5 minutes. Add the tomatoes and brown over medium heat for a few minutes. Remove from the pan and set aside.

Spoon ⅓ cup of the vodka sauce into an 8-inch-square baking pan. Add a layer of eggplant slices and cover with a layer of the tomato-garlic mixture and a layer of the shredded mozzarella cheese. Repeat to make 3 layers, finishing with a layer of vodka sauce.

Sprinkle with the Parmesan, cover with aluminum foil, and bake for 40 minutes. Remove from the oven and let stand at least 10 minutes before cutting and sprinkling with the dehydrated eggplant for added crunch.

Guacamole with Homemade Baked Chips

Growing up, I'd always believed that guacamole was fattening. It wasn't until I discovered that even though its key ingredient, avocado, has fat, it's good fat. I didn't know there were good fats and bad fats, but there are. We all need some fat, not only for flavor but also because your body needs it to function, just like a Ferrari needs oil. My go-to good fats are olive oil; canola oil for cooking; grapeseed oil for salads; almond oil or truffle oil in moderation for flavor; and—of course—avocado.

I love this guacamole with my own homemade baked tortilla chips.

MAKES 4 SERVINGS

3 ripe avocados (not soft and flabby but not six-pack hard, either)

2 garlic cloves

1 shallot

1 jalapeño pepper

½ small white onion, finely chopped

1 lime

Fine sea salt

Handful cilantro, finely chopped

½ ripe tomato, seeded and diced

Paprika, for garnish

Baked corn tortilla chips*

Scoop out the flesh of the avocado. Grate the garlic and shallot; you want the flavor of the juice. If you don't like things too hot, seed the jalapeño pepper, then dice the pepper. (Be careful: don't rub your eyes after handling the pepper until you've washed your hand thoroughly.)

Combine the avocado, grated garlic and shallot, the diced jalapeño, and the chopped onion in a bowl. Squeeze the lime over all and stir to combine. Season with sea salt to taste. Stir in the chopped cilantro, and scatter the tomato over all.

Garnish with the paprika and serve with tortilla chips.

make your own taquitos

Use your home-baked taco chips to make delicious bite-size snacks. Finely chop cooked chicken breast or shrimp, or use cooked ground beef, and combine it in a bowl with diced red onion, tomato, and avocado. Mix the ingredients well, season with salt and pepper to taste, and top each chip with a teaspoonful of the mixture for tasty taquitos pequeños.

*To make your own tortilla chips, spray a baking pan with nonstick cooking spray. Cut corn tortillas into triangles and spread them in the pan. Sprinkle with olive oil, sea salt, and paprika and bake in a 350-degree oven for about 15 minutes, or until crispy.

Breads and Desserts

Mom's Irish Soda Bread

My mom, Lesley Killoren, is smart (she graduated Phi Beta Kappa from Loyola University Chicago), was one of the first American Airlines stewardesses, and she is a great cook who has always been weight conscious. To tell the truth, she never really liked to cook, but I think that was really because she hated the cleanup. On Sunday mornings, however, she often made this Irish soda bread. I got to sleep in on Sundays because there were no swim meets, and the whole family would sit down together for breakfast. My dad, who is of German and Irish descent, loved the bread, and also loved using our breakfasts as vehicles for lecturing us about friends or school. We'd recap what we'd done on Saturday night. My sister usually had something fun to talk about while for me it was often recapping the plot of *The Love Boat*. But no matter what we were saying, somehow Mom always found a way to jump in and turn the subject to sex. It's true! My mom often provided us with a short course in sex education.

I still love Irish soda bread even though I haven't yet figured out how to use it as a platform for talking to my daughters about sex. One of the great things about it, aside from how delicious it tastes, is that a ½-inch-thick slice has only 170 calories!

1½ cups buttermilk

2 tablespoons unsalted butter, melted

1 large egg, slightly beaten

1½ cups dark seedless raisins

3 cups all-purpose flour

⅔ cups sugar

1 tablespoon double-acting baking powder

1 teaspoon baking soda

1 teaspoon fine sea salt

Preheat the oven to 350° F. Grease a 9-by-5-inch loaf pan.

In medium bowl, combine the buttermilk, butter, egg, and raisins; set aside.

In a large bowl, combine the dry ingredients by tossing them together with 2 forks for about 1 minute.

Add the buttermilk mixture to the dry ingredients and mix until combined.

Spoon the batter into the prepared pan and bake for 50 to 55 minutes.

Remove from the oven and leave in the pan for 1 minute. Remove from the pan and cool completely on a wire rack.

The bread is best when freshly baked, so store it wrapped airtight and try to eat it within a day or two.

Where's the Zucchini? Bread

When I was growing up I was a kind of Peter Rabbit. I spent a lot of time stealing vegetables and flowers from our neighbors' garden in Lake Geneva, Wisconsin. But even kids who say they "hate" vegetables will love this bread—and so will you.

MAKES TWO 8-INCH LOAVES;
ABOUT 16 SLICES PER LOAF

3 cups cornmeal

1 teaspoon fine sea salt

1 teaspoon baking soda

3 teaspoons baking powder

3 teaspoons ground cinnamon

3 large egg whites

1 cup grapeseed oil

2¼ cups sugar

3 teaspoons pure vanilla extract

1 small zucchini, shredded

1 small zucchini, finely chopped

Preheat the oven to 325° F. Grease and flour two 8-by-4-inch loaf pans.

Sift the cornmeal, salt, baking soda, baking powder, and cinnamon together into a bowl.

Beat the egg whites, oil, sugar, and vanilla together in a large bowl. Add the sifted ingredients to the egg white mixture, and beat well. Stir in the zucchini until well combined and pour the batter into the prepared pans.

Bake for 40 to 60 minutes until a toothpick inserted in the center comes out clean. Cool in the pans on a wire rack for 20 minutes.

Kiki's Cocoa Crunch

In my mom's defense, she had three kids and it was easier to make the sandwiches for our school lunch the night before, freeze them, and let them thaw in the morning. Except that they never thawed. So I mixed cocoa powder and cereal together and took the mixture to school in plastic baggies for my lunch. Now, instead of a meal replacement, this is my go-to chocolate crunch munch.

MAKES 9 SERVINGS

2 ½ cups organic rolled oats

1 ½ cups unsweetened cereal (any grain or flake)

¼ cup brown sugar

½ cup unsweetened cocoa powder

½ cup maple syrup

1 tablespoon vanilla extract

Organic nonstick cooking spray

Preheat the oven to 250°F and move the rack to the bottom third of the oven.

In a large bowl, combine the rolled oats, cereal, brown sugar, and cocoa powder and mix well. Stir in the maple syrup and vanilla extract until everything is evenly coated.

Spray a large baking sheet with the cooking spray. Spread the mixture evenly over the baking sheet and bake in the preheated oven for one hour.

Cool, break into pieces if necessary, store in baggies, and have it handy for a sweet snack.

Preserve in an airtight jar or container or in Ziploc bags for snacking.

Katharine Hepburn's Brownies

This recipe was my first adventure into baking. I remember it as printed in a newspaper, and it is apparently one of Katharine Hepburn's family recipes. I have always admired Ms. Hepburn for being a pioneer in acting and in fashion. She wore pants and even jeans in 1939. She was *so* cool, and her brownies are amazing!

MAKES 8 BROWNIES

8 tablespoons (1 stick) unsalted butter*

2 squares unsweetened chocolate

1 cup sugar

2 large eggs

½ teaspoon pure vanilla extract

¼ cup all-purpose flour

¼ teaspoon fine sea salt

Preheat the oven to 325°F. Butter and flour an 8-inch-square baking pan and set aside.

In a saucepan over low heat, melt together the butter and chocolate.

Remove from the heat and stir in the sugar, eggs, and vanilla and beat well to combine. Stir in the flour and salt.

Transfer the batter to the prepared pan and bake for about 40 minutes, or until a toothpick inserted in the center comes out clean.

Cool in the pan and then cut into squares.

You can eat these right out of the pan if you want, but it's much nicer to cut them into squares and pile them on a fancy plate. If you want to smarten up your act you can serve them on individual plates with a dollop of *crème fraîche* and a scattering of shaved chocolate.

---

*Unless a recipe specifies salted butter, you should always use unsalted, especially in baking. I always use unsalted butter in all my cooking because it allows me to control how much salt I put in my food.

Mom's Chocolate Cake– aka The Chocolate Devil

My mom's been making this cake since I was a kid. It's always been the bane of her existence and now it's become my nemesis, too. I think she got it from a magazine, but she made her own notes on the torn-out page and adjusted some of the ingredients. For some reason it's devilishly hard to get it right, but when you do it's worth all the fuss because it's the most delicious cake on the planet. Try it on Sunday Funday and start to make some family memories of your own.

MAKES ABOUT 10 SERVINGS

3 squares unsweetened baker's chocolate

2 cups sugar

8 tablespoons (1 stick) unsalted butter

2 large eggs

¾ cup sour cream

1 tablespoon baking soda

2 cups self-rising flour

½ cup water

Preheat the oven to 350° F. Lightly grease a sheet pan or two 8-inch-round cake tins.

In a double boiler over hot, not boiling water, melt the chocolate with 1 cup of the sugar. Set aside to cool.

Using an electric mixer, cream the butter with the remaining 1 cup sugar. Beat in the eggs.

In a small bowl, mix the sour cream with the baking soda and let it stand for a minute, then add it to the batter.

Beat in the flour. Add the water and the cooled melted chocolate mixture and mix well.

Transfer the batter to the prepared pan(s) and bake in the preheated oven for 25 minutes or until a toothpick inserted in the center comes out clean.

Cool in the pan(s) before turning out to cool completely.*

don't be afraid to make it up as you go along

On Season 4 of the *Real Housewives of New York City,* I made a mixed fruit pie for my kids with what was left over in the fruit bowl. I'd never had warm cantaloupe before, but it actually tasted delicious. Don't be afraid to try new things, make mistakes, and have fun doing it. Most of all, don't worry about what other people think about what you like. Who knows, maybe you'll stumble across your own version of a mixed fruit pie. (And don't be afraid to use a store-bought crust.)

*If you are making a layer cake, fill and frost it with your favorite chocolate cake frosting or whipped cream.

Graham Cracker Icebox Napoleons

This is my version of the classic ice box cake made with chocolate wafers.* It is slightly less caloric than a traditional napoleon but not exactly diet fare so save it for Sunday Funday or a special occasion. I like to say I've slimmed Napoleon down a bit and given him some height.

MAKES 4 SERVINGS

24 graham cracker squares

1 pint heavy cream, whipped

1 pint fresh ripe strawberries, hulled and cut in half lengthwise

Place two cracker squares side by side on each of four dessert plates. Spread one-eighth of the whipped cream on top. Scatter one-eighth of the strawberries over the cream. Top with 2 more crackers, another layer of cream and strawberries, and top with the last of the crackers.

make your own ices

Raspberry, mango, strawberry, lychee, pineapple, honey, or lemon teas, or even sweetened espresso, can be frozen to make fabulous homemade ices. Pour into an ice cube tray and stir once or twice during freezing to make it the consistency of a granita.

*The recipe can be increased to make as many servings as you like or to make each napoleon even taller. You can also make it as one big "cake" rather than single servings.

Beverages

GIN-Ginger Beertail

This drink was originally made with gin, but I don't like serving gin drinks because I think it makes people mean. Try it with gin if you dare—just be prepared for a fight.

MAKES 2 DRINKS

2 ounces ginger vodka

2 ounces ginger beer

1 ounce freshly squeezed tangerine juice

3 muddled fresh mint leaves

Dash of sugar

Combine all of the ingredients in a cocktail shaker and use those arm muscles to shake it up. Pour into 2 glasses over ice and enjoy the fruits of your labor.

Kellade

I've always loved both beer and margaritas. So when I was in Mexico and discovered a frozen beer margarita it was like a dream come true. The one I make for myself isn't frozen but it combines three of my favorite things—tequila, beer, and Mexico!

MAKES 1 TALL DRINK

1 ounce Patrón or other high-end Tequila

3 ounces Corona beer

4 ounces lemonade

Juice of ½ lemon

Dash of sugar

Combine all of the ingredients in a cocktail shaker and shake well. Pour into a tall, ice-filled glass and enjoy.

try a frozfruit margarita

For a fun margarita combine a jigger of tequila with a FrozFruit bar of your choice (sans stick, of course) and ice in a blender and blend until smooth. For a party get a selection of different fruit flavors and let your guests pick their favorites.

Babylove

When my oldest daughter was a baby I'd give her a nighttime bottle of formula with a little cereal and banana. As she got older, I began to make her these tasty, healthy shakes.

MAKES 1 DRINK

½ banana, cut up or ½ cup fresh blueberries

6 ounces unsweetened coconut milk

1 tablespoon slivered almonds

1 teaspoon pure vanilla extract

3 to 4 ice cubes

Combine all of the ingredients in a blender and blend until smooth.

Kelly Green Juice

8 fresh mint leaves, chipped

4 fresh lemon balm or parsley leaves, chopped

3 kale leaves, chopped

1 cup chopped broccoli

1 teaspoon freshly squeezed lime juice

½ cup freshly squeezed orange juice

1 cup water

Combine all of the ingredients in a blender and blend until smooth.

Blueberry Lemonade

This is a great nonalcoholic summer cooler, but if you're feeling frisky by all means add the vodka.

MAKES 1 DRINK

6 ounces cold water

Juice of 1 lemon

1 teaspoon cinnamon-sugar, store-bought or make your own with ⅔ sugar and ⅓ cinammon

¼ cup fresh blueberries

3 to 4 ice cubes

1 ounce vodka (optional)

Combine all of the ingredients in a blender and blend until smooth.

Pour into a tall glace, with or without ice cubes.

Kelly's Pink Lemonade

If you'd rather eat your lemonade for dessert, freeze the mixture in ice cube trays to make pink lemonade ices. Or add a jigger of vodka for Perky Pink Lemonade.

MAKES 1 DRINK

6 ounces lemonade

¼ cup fresh raspberries

¼ cup hulled and halved fresh strawberries

Ice cubes

Lime wedge for garnish

Combine the lemonade, raspberries, and strawberries in a blender and blend until smooth. Pour over ice in a tall glass and garnish with the lime wedge.

Superspicy Frozen Margarita

The ultimate in combining sugar and spice!

2 ounces tequila, preferably Patrón

½ jalapeño pepper, seeded and minced*

Juice of 2 limes

Splash of freshly squeezed orange juice

3 to 4 ice cubes

Sugar, for rimming the glass

Combine all of the ingredients except for the sugar in a blender and blend until smooth. Dip the rim of a large martini glass in water, then into the sugar. Pour the drink into the sugar-rimmed glass.

*Leave the seeds in if you dare—they make the drink even *hotter*.

Gummi Bear Martini

If you don't have a paper umbrella handy, Gummi Bears are a great way to put more fun in your drink.

MAKES 1 DRINK

2 parts orange, grape, or other-flavored vodka

1 part Triple Sec

1 part white grape juice

Splash of cranberry juice

Gummi Bears, as many as you like

Combine the vodka, Triple Sec, grape juice, and cranberry juice in a tall glass. Add ice and fill the glass with Gummi Bears.

index

Bad Girl Wings, 183
balance, 26, 34, 45
bananas:
    Babylove, 246
    Extra-Easy Oatmeal, 141
    grilled, 132
    Gr-r-r-anola, 148
    Iguana I Wanna— Cornmeal
      Pancakes, 144–45
    My Favorite Pancakes, 142–43
    So Smooth Smoothie, 146–47
barley:
    Barley Without the Bullfight, 222
    Pencil-Thin Skirt Steak, 172–73
Bar No-Pitti Pasta, 208–9
Bar Pitti, 208
basil:
    Michael Ferraro's Chilled Angel
      Hair Pasta with Garlic, Tomato,
      Basil, and Parmesan, 214–15
    Pasta with Oddkavodka Sauce,
      212–13
beans, 81
    Black Beans and Rice, 220–21
    Warm Quinoa Salad, 162–64
beauty:
    eyes, 100, 101, 116
    hair, see hair
    makeup, 100, 101, 103, 104–8
    must-haves, 118
    plan for, 22
    skin, see skin
    teeth, 111
beef:
    Grilled Rib Eye with Herbes de
      Provence, 170–71
    Mexican Dancer Tortillas, 197

    Pencil-Thin Skirt Steak, 172–73
    Vogue Salad, 166–67
beer, 18–19
Beet Salad, Kelly, 156
Bensimon, Gilles, 6, 7–8, 27, 42–44,
54, 92, 126, 170, 209
beverages:
    Babylove, 246
    Blueberry Lemonade, 248
    GIN-Ginger Beertail, 244
    Gummi Bear Martinis, 251
    Kellade, 245
    Kelly Green Juice, 247
    Kelly's Pink Lemonade, 249
    Superspicy Frozen Margarita, 250
Black Beans and Rice, 220–21
blood sugar, 57–58
blueberries:
    Baby Lamb Chops with Blueberry-
      Mint Salad, 174–75
    Babylove, 246
    Blueberry Lemonade, 248
    Extra-Easy Oatmeal, 141
    My Favorite Cereal, 138–39
    So Smooth Smoothie, 146–47
body type, 94, 96–98
Bowties and Green Pearls, 211
breads:
    Mom's Irish Soda Bread, 232–33
    Where's the Zucchini? Bread,
      234–35
breakfast, 48, 49, 53, 55–56
    Extra-Easy Oatmeal, 141
    Gr-r-r-anola, 148
    Iguana I Wanna— Cornmeal
      Pancakes, 144–45
    My Favorite Cereal, 138–39

Superspicy Frozen Margarita, 250
supplements, 72
sweeteners, artificial, 78
sweet potatoes:
    Crazy Crushed Potatoes, 216
        Yummy Yams, 217

T

tacos, 195
    Shrimp Taco Tuesdays, 194–95
    Tuna Tacos, 198–99
Talbot, Sam, 182
taquitos, 229
Teen, 5
teeth, 111
tempeh burritos, 189
Theodora and Callum, 101
Thursday, 75–90
tilapia, 199, 201
tofu:
    Me Love You Springtime Noodles,
        210–11
    Seth Levine's Pad Thai, 207
tomatoes:
    Eggplant Lasagna, 226–27
    Malibu Chicken Wraps, 182
    Michael Ferraro's Chilled Angel
        Hair Pasta with Garlic, Tomato,
        Basil, and Parmesan, 214–15
    Pasta with Oddkavodka Sauce,
        212–13
    Pizza Mexican Style, 204
tortillas, 195
    Guacamole with Homemade
        Baked Chips, 228–29
    Mexican Dancer Tortillas, 197

Pizza Mexican Style, 204
    Shrimp Taco Tuesdays, 194–95
truffle oil, 20, 228
Tuesday, 25–37
Tuna Tacos, 198–99
turkey:
    clean and neat Joanna, 187
    Christmas Salad, 159
Twitter, 8

V

vegetables, 58
    grilled, 132
    Jimmy Achoo's Chicken Soup,
        150–51
    Seth Levine's Pad Thai, 207
    Spicy Sultry Shrimp and Mango
        Stir-Fry, 190–91
    stuffing and, 51
vitamins, 72
Vogue Salad, 166–67

W

Warm Quinoa Salad, 162–64
water, 37, 45, 57, 77, 84
watermelon:
    grilled, 132
    Supermodel Salad, 155
    wacky, 158
    Watermelon Salad, 158
web sites, 86–89
Wednesday, 39–73
weight, 41
    "freshman fifteen," 34–35
    obesity, 4